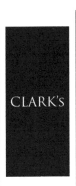

CLARK's

ESSEN

PACS, RIS AND
IMAGING
INFORMATICS

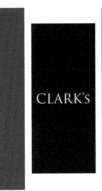

CLARK's

ESSENTIAL PACS, RIS AND IMAGING INFORMATICS

Alexander Peck
LL.M, MSc, BSc (Hons), DipHE, MCP, CITP (BCS)
Superintendent Radiographer & Radiographers Informatics
Training Lead
Communications Lead: BIR Clinical Intelligence & Informatics
Special Interest Group
Chair: SCoR IM+T Advisory Group
Vice President: UK Radiological Congress (Informatics)

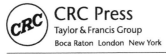

CRC Press
Taylor & Francis Group
Boca Raton London New York

CRC Press is an imprint of the
Taylor & Francis Group, an **informa** business

CRC Press
Taylor & Francis Group
6000 Broken Sound Parkway NW, Suite 300
Boca Raton, FL 33487-2742

© 2018 by Taylor & Francis Group, LLC
CRC Press is an imprint of Taylor & Francis Group, an Informa business

No claim to original U.S. Government works

Printed on acid-free paper

International Standard Book Number-13: 978-1-138-29570-4 (Hardback)
International Standard Book Number-13: 978-1-4987-6323-3 (Paperback)

Visit the Taylor & Francis Web site at
http://www.taylorandfrancis.com

and the CRC Press Web site at
http://www.crcpress.com

For R, B, and C Peck

and

our fellow radiographers making a difference to patient care every hour of every day.

CONTENTS

FOREWORD

This new textbook in the field of imaging informatics is a welcome addition to the Clark's series of pocket and desk-top books. This series is a continuation and tribute to the original work of K C Clark, which now has produced the 13th edition of *Clark's Positioning in Radiography* together with a number of essential specialist reference books.

Miss Clark, I am sure, would welcome this important and comprehensive guide to the modern imaging department, which now at its heart depends on the correct and efficient use of digital imaging technology.

Historically, the darkroom was central to the running of the X-ray department. Today, that role is filled by 'imaging informatics' – without it a modern imaging department would be at a significant disadvantage. This book provides valuable information and guidance as to how imaging informatics for the working radiographer is structured and executed, and will form the basis for providing a safe and efficient environment in which to acquire, store, transfer, and share images with corresponding reports and the valuable patient data.

A Stewart Whitley
Series Editor
Radiology Advisor
UK Radiology Advisory Services
Preston, Lancashire, UK

PREFACE

Running the largest non-profit training programme for imaging informatics in the UK, one of the most frequently received requests has been to collate the many and diverse aspects of the field into a single accessible text.

Imaging informatics itself is a complex and historically rapidly changing field. As a result, this book is intended to be a stepping stone for radiographers, students, assistant practitioners, helpers, and other allied health professionals into the world of imaging informatics by providing a grounding in the basic components of the field. This text covers much ground and rather than being a lengthy be-all-and-end-all of informatics, particularly for the more technical arenas around health level 7 (HL7) and digital imaging and communications in medicine (DICOM), aims to provide a strong foundation for learning in the areas of the readers' choice. While historically taking a back seat in Radiology departments, imaging informatics is today simply a sub-speciality of a well-functioning Radiology department, and here we aim to present informatics in the same manner as those other introductory texts for the more traditional and established modalities.

Suggestions for improvement in future editions, feedback, and corrections are welcome, sent directly to the author at: bookfeedback@pacsgroup.org

Alexander Peck

CONTRIBUTORS

Gareth Baxendale
Head of Technology
NHS National Institute for
    Health Research (NIHR)

Jamie Beck
Lecturer of Diagnostic Imaging
University of Bradford

Oliver Bourached
Informatics Test Lead
Central and North West London
    NHS Foundation Trust

Richard Horton
Service Delivery Manager
NHS National Institute for
    Health Research (NIHR)

Steven Jessop
Business Manager for Sharing
    Solutions
Burnbank Systems Ltd

Anand Patel
Trauma & Orthopaedic Surgeon
Basildon and Thurrock
    University Hospitals NHS
    Foundation Trust

Anant Patel
Informatics Test Team
Central and North West London
    NHS Foundation Trust
and IM+T Advisory Group
    Member Society and College
    of Radiographers

Priya Patel
Solicitor and Director
Legal Eye Compliance and Risk

Rachel Peck
Human Resources Manager
UK Civil Service

Kevin Tucker
National Officer for Wales
Society and College of
    Radiographers

Andrew Ward
Senior Diagnostic Imaging
    Advisor
NHS Wales

Jeremy Weldon
Consultant Reporting Radiographer
London North West Healthcare
    NHS Foundation Trust

Sophie Willis
Senior Lecturer of Diagnostic
    Imaging
City University

Bethan Wyn Owen
Research Radiographer (former
    Directorate Manager)
Betsi Cadwaladr Health Board

ACKNOWLEDGEMENTS

With input from and thanks to: The Society and College of Radiographers IM+T Advisory Group; The British Institute of Radiology Clinical Intelligence & Informatics Committee; The British Computer Society Health Executive; BCS Law; ITSMF UK; Dr Sophie Willis and Darren Walls (Senior Lecturers) of City University School of Radiography; Professor Paul Clough (Professor in Information Retrieval) and Professor Peter Bath (Professor of Health Informatics) of The University of Sheffield Information School; Professor Maryann Hardy (Professor of Radiography and Imaging Practice Research) of the University of Bradford; Bruce Barton (Clinical Specialist Reporting Radiographer), Yousef Mebrate (Medical Engineering and Cardiology Systems Manager) and Christine Peacock (Radiology Services Manager) of the Royal Brompton and Harefield NHS FT; Brandon Bertolli (PACS and Forensic Radiography Freelance Consultant); Rodnick Vassallo (Head of Radiography, former PACS Manager) of St. George's Healthcare NHS Trust; Dr Kate Spacey (Specialist Surgical Registrar) of QE Hospital King's Lynn NHS Trust; Dr Gavin Spence (Consultant Paediatric Orthopaedic Surgeon) of Great Ormond Street Hospital for Children NHS FT; Jane Rendall (UK Managing Director) of Sectra UK and Johan Carlegrim (Cross-Enterprise Product Manager) of Sectra Medical Systems Sweden.

Special thanks to: the fantastic contributing authors, the proof-readers, and reviewers, plus, as always, my personal gratitude to: Adham Nicola (Radiology Systems Manager) and Neil Barron (Superintendent Radiographer for PACS) of London North West Healthcare NHS Trust for their unwavering support, enthusiasm, and endeavours across the years, together with Dr Rhidian Bramley (Chief Clinical Information Officer and Consultant Radiologist) of The Christie NHS FT for his long encouragement; Dr Jason Oakley (Associate Dean) now of the University of Portsmouth for his work in the early millennium, which originally brought me to this speciality; plus Anant Patel and Kevin Tucker for their extensive reviewing, time, and widespread input into our shared goal of promoting radiographer's informatics education.

The contributing authors wish to add their gratitude to Jyotsna Patel.

Supplier acknowledgements

Owing to its inherently costly nature to develop, innovation in imaging informatics is generally driven by the ideas and provisions of supplier software developers. Acknowledgements are given to the assistance from the following organisations: Sectra (who have enthusiastically supported the nationwide programme of vendor-neutral radiographer's imaging informatics education in the UK for over a decade); plus Marval Software, Barco, NEC, Agfa-Gevaert, Pukka-J, Insignia, and GE.

ABOUT THE AUTHOR

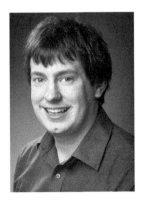

Alexander Peck is the lead for a national non-profit radiographers training team and promotes education in imaging informatics internationally.

Qualified as a diagnostic radiographer, Alexander began working with informatics as a Senior Radiographer at the North West London Hospitals NHS Trust, followed by several years as the former Information Systems Manager at the Royal Brompton & Harefield NHS Foundation Trust.

He is the director of a medical informatics consultancy firm and organiser of the highly popular national non-profit informatics education programme for radiographers and PACS professionals.

Alexander now concentrates on training, the enhancement of cross-enterprise sharing solutions, teaching and research, promoting imaging informatics education and continuing to champion a research-based approach to further developing the better integration of informatics into clinical practice. Awarded Chartered IT Professional status by the British Computer Society, he is Chair of the SCoR IM+T Advisory Group, Communications Lead for the BIR Clinical Intelligence & Informatics Special Interest Group and the current Vice President of the UK Radiological Congress representing informatics.

Alexander is an external lecturer for City University, London, and speaks widely at informatics-related events throughout the country.

ABBREVIATIONS

3D	*three-dimensional*
A&E	*Accident and Emergency (department)*
ACR	*American College of Radiology*
ADT	*admit, discharge, or transfer*
AET	*application entity title*
AHP	*allied health professional*
API	*application program interface*
AQP	*any qualified provider*
ARI	*access to radiology information (IHE)*
AVI	*audio video interleaved*
BC	*business continuity*
BPPC	*basic patient privacy consent (IHE)*
BTU	*British thermal unit*
CAB	*Change Advisory Board*
CAD	*computer aided diagnosis*
CAG	*Change Advisory Group*
CALs	*client access licences*
CCFL	*cold cathode fluorescent lamp*
CCNA	*Cisco certified network associate*
CCNP	*Cisco certified network professional*
CD	*compact disk*
CDSS	*clinical decision support system*
CDS/OAT	*clinical decision support/order appropriate tracking*
CHI	*Community Health Index (Scottish national identifier)*
CIS	*clinical information system (e.g. RIS and LIMS)*
COTS	*commercial off-the-shelf*
CPD	*continuing professional development*
CPOE	*computerised physician order entry*
CR	*computed radiography*
CSP	*cloud service provider*
CT	*computed tomography*
DDR	*direct digital radiography*
DICOM	*digital imaging and communications in medicine*
DMWL	*dynamic modality worklist*

DNA	*did not attend*
DNS	*domain name system*
DPs	*display protocols (also referred to as hanging protocols)*
DPA	*Data Protection Act*
DR	*disaster recovery*
DRL	*diagnostic reference levels*
DTI	*desktop integration*
DVD	*digital versatile disk*
DVI-A	*digital visual interface – analogue output only*
DVI-D	*digital visual interface – digital output only*
DVI-I	*digital visual interface – combined digital and analogue output*
EA	*enterprise archive*
ECG	*electrocardiogram*
EDM	*electronic document management*
EHR	*electronic healthcare record (cradle to the grave record)*
EPR	*electronic patient record*
EU	*European Union*
FAQ	*frequently asked questions*
FHIR	*Fast Healthcare Interoperability Resources (an iteration of HL7)*
FoIA	*Freedom of Information Act*
Gb	*gigabyte*
GDPR	*General Data Protection Regulation*
GM	*general microscopy*
GP	*general practitioner*
HCP	*healthcare professional (radiographer/radiologist/nurse/ GP, etc.)*
HCPC	*Health and Care Professions Council*
H&C	*health and care*
HD	*high definition*
HDD	*hard disk drive*
HDMI	*high definition multi-media interface*
HEI	*higher educational institution*

HIE	*health information exchanges*
HIS	*hospital information system*
HL7	*health level 7*
IaaS	*infrastructure as a service*
ICO	*Information Commissioner's Office*
ID	*identifier*
IDS	*intrusion detection system*
IEP	*image exchange portal*
IG	*information governance*
IGTE	*Information Governance Training Environment*
IHE	*integrating the healthcare enterprise*
IHI	*Individual Healthcare Identifier (Australia)*
ILM	*Institute of Leadership and Management*
IO	*intraoral*
I/P	*in-patient*
IP	*imaging plate/internet protocol (usually suffixed by – address)*
IPEM	*Institute of Physics and Engineering in Medicine*
IR(ME)R	*Ionising Radiation (Medical Exposure) Regulations*
IRR	*Ionising Radiations Regulations*
ISB	*International Standards Board*
ISO	*International Standard Organisation*
IT	*information technology*
ITIL®	*Information Technology Infrastructure Library*
ITSMF	*IT Service Management Forum*
ITT	*invitation to tender*
LAN	*local area network (intranet)*
IVU	*intravenous urography*
JPEG	*Joint Photographic Experts Group*
LCD	*liquid crystal display*
LED	*light emitting diode*
LIMS	*laboratory information management system*
mACM	*mobile alert communications management (IHE)*
MCP	*Microsoft certified professional*

MCITP	*Microsoft certified IT professional*
MDT	*multidisciplinary team (meeting)*
MG	*mammography*
MOD	*magneto-optical disk*
M_o_R®	*Management of Risk*
MPI	*master patient index*
MPR	*multi-planar reconstruction*
MPPS	*modality performed procedure step*
MR(I)	*magnetic resonance (imaging)*
MRZ	*machine readable zone*
MSP	*Managing Successful Programmes*
NACS	*National Administrative Code Service (note: now renamed ODS)*
NAS	*network attached storage*
NBSP	*National Breast Screening Programme*
NBSS	*National Breast Screening Service*
NEMA	*National Electrical Manufacturers Association*
NHI	*National Health Index (Number, New Zealand)*
NHS	*National Health Service (in the UK)*
NICIP	*National Interim Clinical Imaging Procedure*
NM	*nuclear medicine*
NPfIT	*National Programme for IT*
OBS	*output based specification*
OCS	*order communication system (erequesting/status/results)*
ODS	*Organisation Data Service (previously known as NACS)*
OHP	*overhead projector*
OJEU	*Official Journal of the European Union*
O/P	*out-patient*
OSI	*open systems interconnection*
P3O	*Portfolio, Programme, and Project Offices*
PaaS	*platform as a service*
PACS	*picture archiving and communication system*
PAS	*patient administration system*

PC	*personal computer*
pdf	*portable document format*
PET/PT	*positron emission tomography*
PHR	*personal health record*
PID	*patient identification*
POR	*patient owned record*
PPOC	*patient plan of care (IHE)*
PQQ	*pre-qualification questionnaire*
PRINCE2®	*Projects in Controlled Environments (version 2)*
PX	*panoramic X-ray*
QA	*quality assurance*
QR	*quick response*
Q/R	*query/retrieve*
RAM	*random access memory*
RAID	*redundant array of inexpensive disks*
REM	*radiation exposure monitoring (IHE)*
RF	*radiofluoroscopy*
RIS	*radiology information system*
RTx	*radiotherapy components*
SaaS	*software as a service*
SCM	*storage commitment*
SCP	*service class provider*
SCU	*service class user*
SFI	*standing financial instruction*
SFIA	*skills for the information age*
SIAM	*service integration and management*
SIEM	*security information and event management*
SLA	*service level agreement*
SM	*slide microscopy*
SMS	*short message service*
SNA	*supplier neutral archive*
SNOMED-CT	*Systematised Nomenclature of Medicine – Clinical Terms*
SOP	*standard operating procedures/service-object pair*

TCP/IP	*transmission control protocol/internet protocol*
TG	*thermography*
TIF	*tagged image file (format)*
UAT	*user acceptance testing*
UC	*unified communications*
UID	*unique identifier*
UPS	*uninterruptable power supply*
US	*ultrasound*
USB	*universal serial bus*
VDU	*visual display unit*
VFM	*value for money*
VGA	*video graphics array*
VLE	*virtual learning environment*
VM	*value multiplicity*
VNA	*vendor neutral archive*
VPN	*virtual private network*
VR	*voice (speech) recognition/virtual reality/value representation*
WAN	*wide area network*
WSI	*whole slide image*
XA	*X-ray angiography*
XC	*external camera photography*
XCA	*cross-community access (IHE)*
XCA-I	*cross-community access for imaging (IHE)*
XD-LAB	*sharing laboratory reports (IHE)*
XDS/XDS-I	*cross-enterprise document sharing (- for imaging) (IHE)*
XPHR	*exchange of personal health record (describes the content and format of summary information extracted from a PHR system for import into an EHR system, and vice versa) (IHE)*

Generic Names

Throughout this book, generic names rather than brand identifiers are used wherever possible. This is simply because a picture archiving and communication system (PACS) is a picture archiving and communication system regardless of whether it is branded IMPAX, IDS7, Vue, Centricity or some other term, in much the same way as for a radiology information system (RIS). Brand names are given where a single supplier is nationally responsible for a large well-known product.

Regional Variations

The National Health Service is organised differently in each of the four countries – Wales, England, Scotland, and Northern Ireland. Owing to this regional variations do apply and, wherever possible, these are indicated within the text.

CHAPTER 1

INFORMATICS IN RADIOLOGY

What is Imaging Informatics?

Radiology services have become increasingly dependent on computers and digital technologies for their routine activities, especially evident from the millennium onwards in a similar way to other areas in healthcare. Imaging informatics is the collective name given to the field of work and combination of technologies that provide the features of a paper-less or paper-lite department. In particular, imaging informatics is concerned as a speciality with the electronic acquisition, storage, and distribution of the text and image data produced and utilised within a diagnostics department (Radiology, Pathology, Cardiology, etc.) for the wider provision of care and benefit to patients. Imaging informatics is a sub-speciality of health informatics, which is itself defined as: 'The knowledge, skills and tools which enable information to be collected, managed, used and shared to support the delivery of healthcare and promote health' (Department of Health, 2002).

History and Development

Within radiology, for almost a century film was the primary method of handling imaging – with transferring and filing being a manual clerical process. From the early 2000s onwards, the move away from film-producing departments towards the integration of more modern electronic methods began to take place. In the UK this was in part related to national incentives and modernisation projects carried out under the umbrella of the previous National Programme for Information Technology, under which it was ensured that every acute National Health Service (NHS) hospital had deployed a picture archiving and communication system (PACS) and radiology information system (RIS), as well as other electronic health applications. Similarly, paper records of studies and reports have also had their processes modernised, with imaging requests being generated through eRequesting (OCS) systems, and reports published as part of each patient's electronic patient record (EPR). With financial and efficiency-based advantages in modernising radiological departments away from the traditional film, chemical, and paper-based practices, the field of imaging informatics continues to grow rapidly and it is here where radiographers, with their clinical skills, can play a vital role.

By looking at two patient journeys, presented below, the breadth of the profession can become clear.

PATIENT 1

Mrs DuVonne, a 37-year-old French national, falls and is taken by ambulance to a London A&E department with a suspected fracture of the left ankle.

Imaging Informatics Involvement in this Patient Pathway

The patient's demographic details will first be entered into the hospital master patient index (MPI) system; then focussing on radiology – she will need an X-ray, with a request for imaging sent electronically via OCS to RIS, the radiographer will create an attendance for this on RIS, which passes details to the modality and image acquisition station. The practitioner (radiographer in most cases) then acquires the images, makes any post-processing changes needed, and commits the images to PACS. The radiologist or reporting radiographer later views the image on a reporting workstation and dictates a report into either PACS (modern systems) or RIS (historic systems) using desktop integration (DTI) to keep the systems synchronised. This report, once validated, passes to the EPR and might well reach the A&E doctor. Meanwhile the images are burned to disk on a compact disk (CD) robot for return to France, and radiological dose information from the examination added to a national dose audit database.

PATIENT 2

Vera, an 81-year-old, attends an out-patient (O/P) computed tomography (CT) appointment with her carer for assessment of her neurological condition after being referred to a specialist centre from a community site.

Imaging Informatics Involvement in this Patient Pathway

Initially an eReferral is made from her local institution: being an O/P, the patient is already registered on the MPI. Radiology receive the referral electronically prior to the patient's attendance (or sometimes by fax or paper form), the Radiology department books this into a RIS making an appointment that is provided to the patient by letter, SMS (text), or phone call. On attending at reception, the worklist on the CT scanner updates with the patient details, the images are acquired, reconstructions are made on a specialist workstation, and a report issued. The report goes back to Vera's general practitioner (GP) electronically and the images are sent via the national image exchange portal (IEP) back to her local hospital for continuing care and any local follow-up necessary.

From even just the two patient journeys described above, we can ascertain the following scale of the imaging informatics world: MPI, EPR, OCS (eRequesting), eReferral, PACS, RIS, modalities (CT, nuclear medicine [NM], magnetic resonance [MR], ultrasound [US], X-ray angiography [XA], direct digital radiography [DDR], computed radiography [CR]...), other hospital applications (billing, dose monitoring), export robots... and of course the hardware, networks, interconnections, and infrastructure that supports all of these. If at any point in the process there is a failure, either patient care will be interrupted or significant delays are introduced into the journey. Cumulatively, over hundreds of patients per day, these delays can be costly and detrimental to the health of those using the services – it is for this reason that imaging informatics plays a vital role in the modern healthcare environment.

Main Components in Radiology

Within radiology, PACS and RIS are the most visible components. Together, these systems work with acquisition modalities to underpin radiology services, handling both the text and data generated in the department. As delays in radiology generally result in a wider delay in patient care, when one or other of the two systems stops working efficiently, knock-on effects are noticeable throughout a hospital within a short space of time. Imaging informatics professionals generally begin their careers in administering these two systems only, then are gradually exposed to the remainder of the profession over time as they gain experience and knowledge.

Data Flows

Between each of these applications, systems, and pieces of machinery is the flow of data. **Fig. 1.1** shows the scale of a typical data flow for a diagnostics service, such as Radiology. Each of these components will be examined in more detail throughout this book.

Bridges (or connections) between applications provide interoperability between systems and are known as 'interfaces'; however, interfaces have the unfortunate reputation for being the 'weak link' in informatics estates. Although interoperability is a corporate goal in many information technology (IT) strategies, reducing the number of interfaces, or at least the number of interfaces required for use in each individual data flow, is the personal goal of many informatics professionals.

Human Factors

Not just a field involved with data, hardware, and software, imaging informatics professionals must also consider human factors in their daily work. The main consideration is digital literacy, which plays a large role in the smooth adoption and correct, efficient use of informatics technologies, and includes examining the use of information, managing digital identities, and understanding the impact of new technologies on existing processes. While many new to the imaging informatics profession may have been exposed throughout their childhood to computers and IT, it must be remembered that a great number of the population were not, and it is important that suitable education

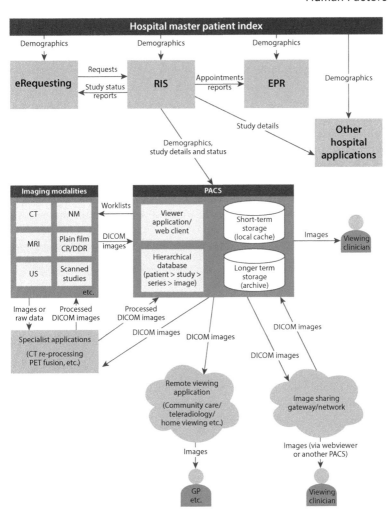

Fig. 1.1 Overview of imaging informatics applications. (CR/DDR, computed radiography/direct digital radiography; CT, computed tomography; DICOM, digital imaging and communications in medicine; EPR, electronic patient record; GP, general practitioner; MRI, magnetic resonance imaging; NM, nuclear medicine; PACS, picture archiving and communication system; PET, positron emission tomography; RIS, radiology information system; US, ultrasound.)

and training programmes are put in place to support these people to ensure they are able to keep pace with developments in the ITs that affect their clinical practice.

Another key human factor to be considered when becoming involved in informatics is the impact of changes on current practice – a common example in healthcare is when users utilising a newly introduced system find they cannot skip or avoid steps that they were able to ignore with paper (mandatory fields being a prime example). Users will then work to prove that the system takes too long and slows down their day-to-day actions, which in turn promotes a negative experience, slowing useful benefit realisation. However, with good engagement, involvement of those in key positions, and wider consultation in advance it would be possible to cascade the reasoning behind certain requirements, resulting in more constructive suggestions being offered.

CHAPTER 2

BASIC IT FOR RADIOGRAPHERS

Components of IT equipment used within the healthcare environment are many and varied. Those frequently part of the informatics estate can be categorised into two distinct types: hardware and software.

Hardware

Workstations/PCs

- *Processor*: the heart of every workstation is a processor. This device in its simplest form takes collections of digital inputs (0 or 1) and processes them into outputs upon the instructions received from the programs currently running. The speed of the processor directly influences the speed the user perceives when using the workstation.
- *Memory*: in this context, random access memory (RAM) is a high-speed place for items currently in use to be stored. The more RAM available, the more items (programs, instructions, user data, etc.) can be used and manipulated at the same time. Applications, such as three-dimensional (3D) reconstructions, require larger amounts of RAM than viewing a single plain radiographic image. Equated to a human task, RAM is equivalent to human short-term memory – some people can remember longer sequences of numbers than others. RAM is measured in gigabytes (Gb).
- *Graphics card*: this is a second processor and extra memory dedicated to displaying images. It is needed owing to the greater complexity of modern applications requiring different mathematical operations than the standard processor is designed for.

- *Storage*: either a hard drive (a spinning magnetic disk) or solid state drive (a miniaturised internal device, similar in principle to a large, fast memory card) where data are stored, even when powered off.

Input/Output Devices

Input/output devices can either be attached to the workstations or personal computers (PCs) by wires (wired devices) or by radio frequency transmissions (wireless). Wireless devices, such as keyboard or mice, have historically had poor levels of security (mostly no security) meaning that keystrokes and movements can be intercepted silently by a malicious eavesdropper in the area. Only devices with strong encryption for their radio communications should be used in a healthcare environment: a reason why wired peripherals are currently preferred.

- *Input devices*:
    - **A mouse** provides navigation of the cursor on-screen. Mice can either be traditional in style (pebble shaped), upright (shaped like an iceberg for those with limited wrist movements), 3D (aka a gyromouse/fitted with a gyroscope for handheld use in theatres or multidisciplinary team (MDT) meetings), projection (a sensor detects hand movements within a fixed area), button (shaped as a 'pencil eraser' and used in a similar manner to a joystick), rollerball (a captive ball, as used in self-check-in kiosks or arcade machines), or presented as a trackpad (flat, with a touch sensitive box). The choice of mouse depends on the nature of the application and its environment.
    - **Keyboards** can incorporate smart card readers and be of many different styles, with or without washable membranes or covers for clinical use and sterilisation.
    - **Foot pedals** are used for inputting shortcuts, traditionally in radiology transcription workflows, but are also useful for those with limited hand movements.
    - **Dictation microphones**: the most commonly used model in the UK is the Philips SpeechMike (various versions), which has a built-in speaker for playback, a trackball, and several

customisable buttons (some used for reporting functions, others for the user's choice).

- **Touchscreen monitors**: either capacitive (using the surface to discharge a tiny electrical current through the user's body) or resistive (a mesh sandwiched between two clear sheets, which closes electrical contacts at specific places on each tap), each giving particular advantages in different situations (resistive screens operate with gloved fingers, capacitive do not if the glove is not conductive).

- *Output devices*:
  - **Displays, printers** (discussed more later).
  - **Speakers:** for playback of audio (listening to original voice files to verify transcription, etc.).

- *Dual purpose devices:*
  - **Memory sticks/CD/digital versatile disk (DVD)/Blu-ray disks and drives:** comparatively low capacity removable media used generally for the physical transfer of images to solicitors or by patients for onward care. Security risks are prevalent with these, as discussed in Chapter 4. These devices could also be used for input purposes.
  - **3.5 inch 'floppy' drives:** obsolete in many uses because of their lack of capacity; however, firmware updates for some CR machines (the raw machine operating instruction coding) still utilise these formats for both input and output owing to the resilience and longevity of the media.
  - **Magneto-optical disks (MODs):** for long-term archival of larger volumes of data, these were historically common for storing unprocessed CT data (the raw output of the scan before processing took place) or older PACS archives, sometimes in large jukebox machines for automated physical storage or retrieval. Again, these may be utilised for both input and output.

Peripherals often connect into ports known as universal serial bus (USB) ports, which are ubiquitous on modern PCs. The USB standard is continually evolving, with many devices in use today utilising version

2 (USB v2) or version 3 (USB v3) if faster transfer rates are required. When the same size connector is used between the versions, USB v3 ports have a blue bar to indicate the availability of the increased speed, which is essential to consider if there are multiple devices to be connected to a mix of version 2 and 3 ports (devices such as removable hard drives should be given first choice of a faster v3 port).

Display Devices

Comprising multiple components, display devices are where the primary output of a PC is displayed to the user. The most visible component(s) of this is one or more monitors (also known as displays, screens or visible display units [VDUs]). Different types of monitors are available depending on the purpose and use of the workstation to which they are attached. High-quality monitors for reporting require dedicated graphics cards to operate – these are specialist processors internal to the workstation in a card shape, which provide the necessary outputs to the monitors. Various types of cabling are used to connect monitors to the graphics cards: the most common high-resolution interfaces being high-definition multimedia interface (HDMI), DisplayPort, digital visual interface (DVI) – digital output only (DVI-D) and combined digital and analogue output (DVI-I). Outdated legacy interfaces included video graphics array (VGA), S-Video, and proprietary interfaces, which may still be in service to connect aged infrastructure in MDT or conference rooms.

The most widely used colour display devices are flat panel monitors with images composed of a grid formed by millions of alternating red, green, and blue pixels, which are backlit by bright white light-emitting diodes (or previously but now less commonly, cold cathode fluorescent tubes). Owing to manufacturing processes, many low-end monitors have a number of 'dead' or 'stuck' pixels even when new. Dead pixels are tiny sections of the screen that do not operate, whereas stuck pixels are tiny areas that are permanently on, displaying their colour. For high quality diagnostic displays, the backlight is manufactured to precision standards, certified to be completely uniform (no areas of high or low brightness) with the number of working pixels being extremely close to 100%. Some new diagnostic displays, e.g. specialist screens for breast tomosynthesis reporting, remain greyscale only and use a liquid crystal matrix to selectively block light in order to maintain the highest pixel density possible (to allow for the reporter to spot tiny calcifications).

Printers

Covering a variety of outputs, three main types of printer are found in imaging departments.

- Plain paper: for appointment letters, documents, printed lists, etc. (standard office laser or inkjet printers, similar to domestic counterparts, but with larger toner/ink capacities).
- Thermal: for labels, stickers, CD/DVD tops or patient wristbands, being either direct thermal (burning the surface of the sticker) or indirect dye sublimation (melting dye from a plastic carrier ribbon to transfer ink onto the surface of the sticker).
- Film: for limited uses, such as patients returning to non-digital healthcare systems abroad. Film printers were previously widely used for business continuity during PACS outages, but are now being depreciated within UK Radiology departments because of the limited shelf life of the film packs used, physical size of the units, and annual maintenance costs involved. As PACS and the supporting hospital infrastructure are now routinely very stable, it is no longer necessary or common for departments to retain film printing technology on-site.

UPS

Uninterruptable power supplies (UPS) provide a temporary source of replacement battery power should mains supply be lost, either accidentally or as part of a planned test. They connect in series between the wall socket and workstation to allow enough time for either the mains power to be restored or for the computer to be shut down gracefully (by saving documents, sending images or completing any reports in progress, etc.). They are recommended for all clinical workstations or devices (including modalities) where abrupt shutdown of a machine would present a clinical risk or disruption to the service. UPS devices traditionally also 'filter' incoming mains power of any harmful spikes in voltage, which may damage the more expensive workstations.

Servers

Servers are the devices that run centralised applications, such as the backend functionality of a PACS or RIS, and in most cases are housed within a dedicated environment managed by the local IT department, known as the server room. Servers are effectively powerful customised workstations and can either be dedicated (known as 'pizza box' servers owing to their shape) or virtual (running as virtual instances on shared hardware). Dedicated pizza box servers are measured in physical size in 'U's, with 1 U being 4.4 cm of height in a standard server rack, with cooling requirements measured in British thermal units (BTUs). An IT department uses the total number of BTUs output by all servers in a given area to calculate the volume of air conditioning required. Within the server room, when adding or updating a dedicated server, considerations include whether there is sufficient power available, sufficient cooling, and whether any infrastructure (network, cabling, physical space) is suitable for the revised requirements. Virtual servers can be measured in many ways, but commonly with processor 'seats' being indicated (the more of these seats, the more 'powerful' the virtual server can be made). As virtual servers can share physical hardware in the server room (and so have lower power, cabling, and cooling requirements), they are commonly preferred by IT departments; however, as PACS and imaging informatics applications have heavy demands on hardware, debate is ongoing as to whether this is the best option, or whether dedicated pizza box servers remain the better choice in the long term, despite the higher physical space, power, and overall cooling requirements. Pizza box servers with associated racks of hard disk storage space are shown in **Fig. 2.1**: a typical 2010's era installation.

Connected to either type of radiology server is typically a storage array, UPS, and backup device to hold all the data being utilised and provide protection.

Networks

Networks provide the physical interconnections and backbone between pieces of IT. A surprising amount of work for the imaging informatics professional originates from the network infrastructure of the healthcare institution (or faults therein!). This provides an incentive for informatics professionals in the field to study network-based training programmes to help them understand the potential problems and configuration options to speed up or increase reliability of

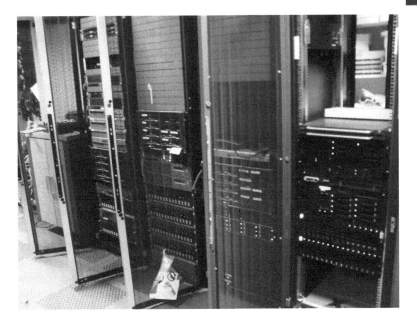

Fig. 2.1 Typical 2010's era radiology systems server racks with hard disk storage arrays. The server racks are housed in perforated metal cages to allow for high air-flow (for cooling).

radiology services. Main components of network infrastructure are the routers and switches with interconnecting cables.

Cabling. The physical make-up of network cabling is either traditional copper (utilising the flow of electrons/electricity) or now the more common glass fibre-based cabling (utilising the flow of photons/light). Glass fibre-based networking has theoretically much higher speeds than that utilising copper owing to the physics behind the two technologies. However, due to the relative newness of the glass fibre-based networking devices, while it is currently commonplace for the 'spine' of a network to utilise this newer technology, the 'final hop' (final connection) to the workstation, server, or device typically remains made in copper cable. This will change over the coming years as the higher raw material cost of copper balances out the higher cost of glass fibre installations, with greater throughput (amounts of data that can be moved around) being the consequence.

Internet protocol addresses. Networks are also on the cusp of another change: addressing the data flowing around a network is much like a telephone or postal system using telephone numbers or post codes. Data to be moved around, such as a webpage or radiology image, is broken down into thousands of tiny 'packets' of data, each containing a destination and technical data. The main 'addressing' system used throughout the world is currently the same as that devised in 1981, namely internet protocol (IP)V4 (where addresses are denoted as blocks of numbers in fixed ranges, such as 192.168.0.1, similar to telephone numbers with area codes). However, as IPV4 has a fixed number of addresses that have now run out (because items such as internet connected mobile telephones, fridges, and closed-circuit TV cameras were not foreseen in the 1980s) a transition to a newer addressing standard, IPV6, is underway. IPV6 uses hexadecimal addresses (fd00:ab4f:4201:abf2:fbc4:f1ac:ba53:abc1), which offer substantially more combinations than with IPV4. There are central 'directories' of IP addresses within both an institution, country, and the world to ensure duplication is minimised on the wider internet, and also to provide routing details.

Routers. These connect several different networks and operate at the network layer (level 3) of the open systems interconnection (OSI) model (see health level 7 [HL7], Chapter 9). These devices can broadcast data packets within an internal intranet network (a local area network: LAN) and outwards into a wide area network (WAN), such as the general internet. Routers typically assign and maintain the local IP addresses and associated directory to machines, workstations, and devices that connect to the network, plus critically the most direct/fastest routes between various points.

Switches. These create a network, operating at the data link layer (level 2) of the OSI model and receive and forward data packets in the internal network only, using the router's instructions.

Port. This is a digital entry or exit point, similar to a real life ferry terminal, bus station, or airport. The de facto port used for unsecure digital imaging and communications in medicine (DICOM) transmission is 104, with secure DICOM passing into the speciality allocated and reserved port 2762.

VPN. A virtual private network (VPN) allows for connections between two normally separate networks to take place, creating a secure 'tunnel' between the two points. Most typically this is observed between a hospital network and the homes of staff – allowing for staff to access internal hospital applications in a secure manner. VPN tunnelling can either be 'full' or 'split'. Full tunnelling should be utilised wherever possible, which directs all traffic (including general internet searches and printer requests) onto the remote network, allowing the user to experience it as if they were in the hospital itself. Split tunnelling directs only specific traffic and is more open to security risks but is cheaper (less traffic load is placed into the remote site).

Bandwidth. This is the amount of data that can be simultaneously sent over a given connection, which is a crucial consideration when a large number of either modalities (perhaps CT scanners) or radiology reporting workstations are situated close together; is there sufficient bandwidth in that area for all the machines planned?

Software

Software plays a supporting role in making best use of the hardware capabilities and is responsible for the interface with which the user interacts. Good interfaces speed up human interaction times and increase productivity.

Operating System

The main component running on any workstation or server – the Microsoft Windows operating system – is traditionally utilised in healthcare environments across the UK. This is collectively for licensing reasons (bulk licensing across the NHS was previously entered into), for the range of applications available owing to the 'openness' of programming tools, the familiarity of the platform to many staff from the domestic environment, and overall the lifetime cost of alternative competing systems.

Active Directory

Local to each healthcare institution or group of institutions within a region, an active directory provides a single point of authentication

Table 2.1 Common destinations of backups

Backup type	Advantages	Disadvantages
Cloud	Flexible sizing; generally more secure because professional data centres are used; comparatively easy to restore if original premises/equipment is destroyed/inaccessible	Loss of internal organisational control (reliance on the outsourced company); reliance on internet/3rd party network; potential security/confidentiality issues if data not encrypted before upload
Tape/MOD	Can be locally managed; directly connected backup hardware is fast	Backup media required to be purchased and maintained; media must be stored in secure, fire/flood proof environment; media curation can be difficult
Mirrored server	If mirrored to another site, possibility to maintain service if original site hardware is damaged; data remain under organisational control	High network bandwidth demands; requires mirrored hardware, with cost and space considerations
NAS	Reasonably fast if using intranet (a private network internal to an organisation); simple, flexible, and comparatively inexpensive destination for backups	If hosted in the same building, risk of physical damage; portable NAS storage has durability issues

MOD, magneto-optical disk; NAS, network attached storage.

for multiple tasks, including Microsoft Windows logon, and logon to various systems including most PACS and RIS.

Backups

A hybrid of hardware and software, undertaking and verifying backups is a common daily task (or chore!) for PACS team members owing to the consequences of losing medical data (which would include re-irradiation of patients if related imaging data were lost). *Table 2.1* details the most common destinations of backups in use at present. Verifying these backups is a frequently missed task for Radiology departments, but is necessary for validating that the backups would be useful in the event of them being called into use.

Table 2.2 What gets backed up and when?

	Full	Incremental	Differential
1st Backup	Entire dataset	Entire dataset	Entire dataset
2nd Backup	Entire dataset	Changes from 1st backup	Changes from 1st backup
3rd Backup	Entire dataset	Changes from 2nd backup	Changes from 1st backup
…	Entire dataset	Changes from previous backup	Changes from 1st backup

Backups can be either full, incremental or differential depending on the chosen backup plan and requirements of the application:

- *Full backups* take the entire dataset (e.g. a RIS database, or a PACS repository) and create an identical copy, either by lossless compression or in raw 1:1 format. This is both time consuming and resource intensive.
- *Incremental backups* include only data that have changed from the previous backup.
- *Differential backups* are similar to incremental backups, but include all data changed from the very first, full backup (rather than a previous differential backup).

The various backup types are illustrated in *Table 2.2*.

Resilience. Some systems make use of identical copies of their hardware, which can 'load balance' (share loading to provide even wear) between each other during normal use, or 'failover' (continuing to use the non-failed components) in the event one piece fails in order to provide redundancy. For storage, a redundant array of inexpensive disks (RAID) can be utilised to give the same resilience for disks (and also performance boosts in some cases). Various 'levels' of RAID provide different amounts of failure tolerance, with RAID 10, e.g. providing data mirroring and striping across multiple disks allowing at minimum one disk out of the 'array' to fail yet the system being able to continue operating with no data loss. RAID only provides resilience and should not be considered a backup solution.

Clinical Digital Maturity Index

The clinical digital maturity index of all hospitals is ranked in the UK based on a number of measureable attributes, such as having the right leadership, infrastructure, and governance regimens in place, as well as how many processes remain paper-based, or paper-lite, rather than being fully digital.

N3

The N3 network, provided by British Telecom, is a secure network connecting the majority of healthcare institutions and providers across the UK. This allows for cross-organisational working without having to establish multiple VPNs criss-crossing the country. The N3 network contains its own national intranet system (webpages on this begin with nww. rather than www.).

NHS.net

General email traffic is unsecure. English and Scottish NHS Trusts, along with many private healthcare providers, utilise a well established, centralised secure email service (a 'white-label' Microsoft Outlook) in order to exchange confidential information securely between different institutions via electronic message. This service is now provided by Accenture (formerly provided by Cable & Wireless until 2016).

IMAGE ACQUISITION

An imaging 'modality' is a term given to a particular type of image acquisition method, such as CR, DDR, US, CT, MR, NM, or radiotherapy components (RTx). The majority of the image acquisition methods communicate images electronically into the PACS using the DICOM standards after the operator has post-processed them.

Regardless of the type, acquisition equipment has six standard functions:

1. Identify the patient and exam.
2. Acquire image(s).
3. Associate image(s) with patient and study data.
4. Provide necessary post-processing features.
5. Transmit the image(s) to a storage location (PACS).
6. Maintain a temporary local database for a short period of time as a business continuity measure (in the event of PACS or network failure).

From an image acquisition point of view, imaging modalities can be split into one of three broad types depending on their output: single image, multi-image, and hybrid modalities. All outputs are initially structured binary data, assembled into a form interpretable by a human.

Single Image Modalities

With imaging modalities such as CR, DDR, US, and even film digitisers, the post-acquisition processing functions may be incorporated into a workstation at the acquiring device and the amount of post-processing

Table 3.1 Single image modalities

DICOM modality code	Modality name	Imaging outputs
CR	Computed radiography	Single images
DX	(Direct) digital radiography	Single images
US	Ultrasound	Single images, which can be collated into stacks
NM	Nuclear medicine	Single images, which can be collated
RF	Radiofluoroscopy	Single images, usually always stacked
XA	X-ray angiography	Single images, possibly stacked or videos
MG	Mammography	Single images
IO	Intraoral radiography	Single images
XC	External camera photography (aka. visible light)	Single images
SM	Slide microscopy	Pathology single images
GM	General microscopy	Pathology single images
OP	Ophthalmic photography	Single images
TG	Thermography	Single images
PX	Panoramic X-ray	Single images
OT	Other	Typically scans of request forms, or scanned historic films

Note: This table utilises the modality codes as listed in the DICOM standard.

is generally routine and less time-consuming (traditionally comprising applying secondary shuttering, annotations, checking layout/positioning, and minor adjustments to image window widths/levels). Angiographic or fluoroscopy equipment also falls into this category, as the motion imaging produced is acquired in a similar manner. Single image modalities are listed in *Table 3.1*.

Multi-Slice Modalities

Multi-slice modalities, which produce complex raw data imaging sets, have separate workstations and applications to allow for the intricate and detailed post-acquisition processing to take place. This is commonly found with CT, MR, and NM imaging modalities, where the

Table 3.2 Multi-slice modalities

DICOM modality code	Modality name	Imaging outputs
CT	Computed tomography	Single images, stacked into multiple series
MR	Magnetic resonance	Single images, stacked into multiple series
ECG	Electrocardiography	Waveforms
RTIMAGE	Radiotherapy image	Single images, stacked into multiple series
RTPLAN	Radiotherapy plan	Single images, stacked into multiple series

Note: This table utilises the modality codes as listed in the DICOM standard.

acquired imaging is re-processed to allow for the clinical question to be answered. The re-processed data are then stored to PACS for future reference and for clinicians outside of radiology to refer to. Popular multi-slice modalities are listed in *Table 3.2.*

Hybrid Modalities

Where two types of imaging acquisition are combined during one examination.

- *PET imaging* utilises combinations of CT, MR and NM to produce a fused image demonstrating both high quality anatomical detail with radioactivity emissivity data.
- *3D volumetric motion imaging* (for functional analysis of joints during movement) draws on the combination of CT and multi-angle visual light recording to generate 3D renderings of the skin and skeletal isosurface for later analysis by physiotherapists or other healthcare professionals involved in rehabilitation.

Core hybrid modalities relevant to imaging informatics professionals are listed in *Table 3.3.*

Specialist Applications

Several modalities now produce complex raw data sets and in many cases it is not efficient from a workflow process perspective to carry out all post-processing at the actual acquisition station. This may be

Table 3.3 Hybrid modalities

DICOM modality code	Modality name	Imaging outputs
PT	Positron emission tomography	Single images, stacked into multiple series (later combined/fused for display and interpretation)
(not issued)	3D volumetric motion imaging	Single images, stacked into multiple series (later combined/fused for display and interpretation)

Note: This table utilises the modality codes as listed in the DICOM standard.

because of time constraints (a room is required for the acquisition of imaging repeatedly or the acquiring member of staff is required to continue with other patients at that time) or skill differences (a member of staff trained in specific image manipulation may be required to carry out the final changes as per the requirements of the reporting process). The manipulations of the imaging described below can then take place after the images have been acquired.

Multi-planar and 3D Reconstructions

By taking raw data from multi-planar modalities, such as CT or MR, almost limitless projections can be generated to best optimise the images for reporting. Multi-planar reconstruction (MPR) facilities are routinely found on workstations attached to the modality in question, but can also be provided in modern image viewers attached to a PACS. 3D rendering takes MPR a step further, allowing for 'real-life' dissections of imaging, removal of obscuring structures (the scan table or head pads, for instance) and colour rendering of structures at pre-set depths to allow for better visual acuity during reporting.

Vessel Analysis and Colon Navigation

Both of these are now gaining in popularity but require advanced graphics processing abilities – effectively the 'pipes' (be they blood vessels or part of the large bowel) are processed in 3D and rendered so that the reviewer can either measure the cross-sections, or 'fly' through them, staying within the bounds of the structure. Until the latter part of the 2010s this type of processing was limited to dedicated workstations, and now many PACS providers include this functionality as an add-on for any suitably powerful PC.

Orthopaedic Templating

Surgical implants are costly. Established in the early 2000s, orthopaedic templating allows for the removal of the manual processes that historically took place in theatres prior to an orthopaedic procedure. Now, instead of holding an overhead projector (OHP) transparency with an outline of the implant options printed on it over a piece of radiographic film, surgeons can annotate images and plan which sizes of implants to utilise in advance, digitally. Although this has minimal impact on the actual imaging departments, it has provided significant time and cost savings to the surgical departments who can now better choose the correct devices rather than working from an approximation (and having to open, then potentially discard any wrong choice of surgical implants). This type of application operates from standard CR or DDR images, but requires calibration. To calibrate, an object of known size must be placed in line with the patient's anatomy in question at the time of imaging. This can be a perfectly spherical ball bearing of known diameter attached either directly or indirectly to patient anatomy – perhaps the lateral aspect of the hip when hip replacements are being considered (**Fig. 3.1**). Spherical ball bearings are used as they have the same dimensions in all directions, unlike a coin or flat disk.

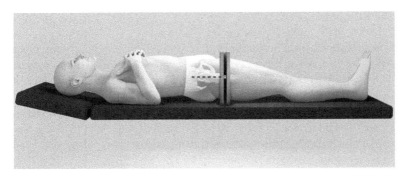

Fig. 3.1 Standard anatomical positioning of orthopaedic templating apparatus.

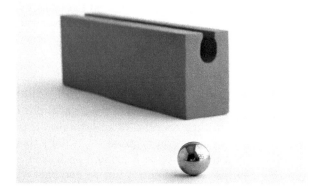

Fig. 3.2 Indirect attachment orthopaedic templating apparatus.

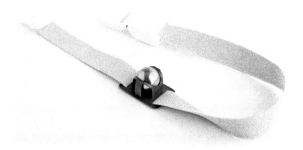

Fig. 3.3 Direct attachement orthopaedic templating apparatus.

These spheres can be supported in a flexible stand, a foam block (**Fig. 3.2**), an elastic holder (**Fig. 3.3**) or, more conveniently and hygienically, stuck to the patient with inexpensive disposable foam rings. It is commonplace to require ball bearings to be placed on all potential orthopaedic images in order to avoid re-irradiating a patient just to acquire an image for templating. Orthopaedic templating modules now widely include the ability to manipulate prosthesis templates and bone fragments identified on radiographs in 3D (**Fig. 3.4**).

After the image post-processing has been completed in any specialist application, the re-processed data can be stored to PACS, alongside the original imaging if required. Some institutions prefer

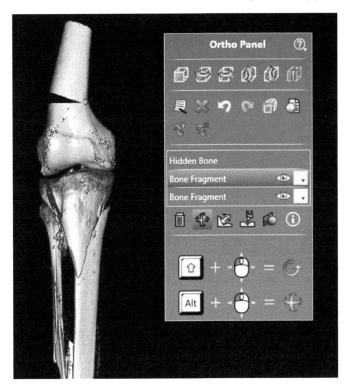

Fig. 3.4 Three-dimensional manipulation of bone fragments during surgical reconstruction planning.

to store reconstructed data to a separate location in order to preserve storage space on the main hospital PACS. In previous years, backups of the re-processed data (and the original raw data acquired) were stored on removable media, such as MODs, and it was not uncommon to see rows of such disks on custom built shelves lining the corridors of CT staff areas; today, these data are either stored to PACS or another dedicated local archive instead.

For a fuller account of how each modality operates individually, refer to the relevant sections in *Clark's Positioning in Radiography*, 13th edition.

Engineering

From an informatics point of view, image acquisition modalities present a challenge, in that when installed they are generally configured by the supplier staff, who are constrained by a deadline. It is therefore good practice for a sheet showing the correct default settings required for integration into the various informatics systems (including examples of acceptable machine names – application entity titles (AETs) – and correct formatting of the institution name, address, etc.) to be made available to all modality superintendents/department heads in order to prevent incorrect settings from having to be rectified later. When tendering or purchasing modalities outright it is recommended that purchasers require suppliers to provide all engineering codes and items necessary to obtain full access to engineering and installation settings as a matter of course – preventing the need for costly and difficult to co-ordinate call-outs to make simple connection changes as is occasionally necessary. This may require the modality suppliers to furnish a service dongle, or simply a list of codes to the PACS Manager or equivalent, updated as necessary.

CHAPTER 4

PACS, VENDOR NEUTRAL ARCHIVES AND PICTURE STORAGE

Picture Archiving and Communication Systems

A PACS is a centralised computer-based system designed to manage healthcare images acquired as part of the examination process via digital image acquisition modalities. It provides the facility for the storage, distribution, and electronic display of the acquired images, supporting clinical diagnostics, improving the patient journey, enhancing clinical care, and allowing for more detailed treatment or follow-up planning.

PACS can be used in any department (not just Radiology), including Cardiology, Pathology, Echocardiography, and Medical photography and for the storage of electrocardiograms (ECGs).

For decades, physical film and chemical processing was used extensively within Radiology departments, with the resultant films being stored in one large cardboard envelope per patient in film archives.

These film archives took up a tremendous amount of physical space, were expensive (traditional radiological film contains silver), a fire hazard, and resulted in a not inconsiderable number of 'lost' films or reports owing to misfiling or loss. To view a film, the patient's film packet had to be first requested from the film library, conveyed to the viewing location, and the films assembled in the order required for viewing – a cumbersome and slow process.

Initially, digital modalities, such as CT or CR, began to store their own images internally; however, it was quickly realised that this was impractical and that there was a need to distribute. Centralised PACS began to be installed, and in the UK early adopters (prior to the millennium), such as the Hammersmith Hospital followed by the Central Middlesex Hospital, provided valuable experiences for the country. PACS was widely understood to bring financial and efficiency gains over historic processes, and this provided a push for the National Programme for IT (NPfIT) to become established by the Department for Health, providing for installation of RIS and PACS across the majority of the NHS (and equivalent health boards) by 2006. In 2017, there are only a small handful of departments utilising film remaining and these are mostly extremely specialist sites, e.g. small dental practices or veterinary clinics.

PACS are highly customisable, and while off-the-shelf packages are available, systems in place in the UK are usually tailored to the particular needs of each healthcare institution. For example, some sites implement varying levels of data compression – where radiological image files are compressed to reduce their storage size and increase their speed of display. The retention period, volume, and type of imaging stored to each PACS is likewise unique to each site, and a decision made jointly by radiologists, imaging staff, and facility management. The types of medical multi-media able to be stored and viewed are similarly unique to each installation.

There are many vendors offering PACS in some form within the UK, the choice being down to the skill level of the PACS team (a higher skilled and experienced PACS team has the option to consider systems requiring greater involvement and levels of customisation, whereas an institution with no PACS team would most likely be better suited to a PACS offering less local configuration and administrative interactivity).

Components

As shown in **Fig. 4.1**, at its core PACS consists of four discrete parts that together include both software and hardware elements.

Short-term storage (local cache). This is a fast short-term storage device; new images sent from acquisition modalities arrive here allowing for rapid viewing of the most recent images.

Longer term storage (archive). This is a longer term storage device, which may comprise online media or offline media. Older images are stored here, with images being copied from the short-term storage after a day or so, with the copy on the short-term storage being deleted from there after a set period (perhaps 6 months), leaving only the copy in the archive.

Viewer application. This is a software program for viewing the images. Viewer applications can also contain additional or advanced features (e.g. slab functionality, MPR, and 3D reconstruction components or specialist imaging analysis tools) to allow for further manipulation and processing of the images. These viewing applications may be installable software, or web-based clients of various types. Typically, there is a single version of the viewer application for all users, or a cut-down version for the majority of users plus an enhanced tailored version for use on dedicated reporting workstations. Dedicated reporting workstations are routinely found in radiology and are comparatively powerful high quality computer hardware, with specialist display monitors.

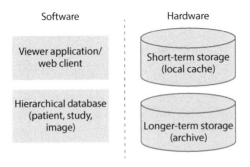

Fig. 4.1 The basic software and hardware components of a generic PACS.

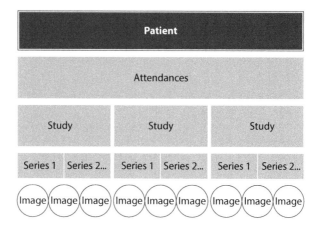

Fig. 4.2 The hierarchical structure of a PACS database.

Hierarchical database. Radiological imaging is organised in a pre-defined and easily determined manner – it produces structured data. At the heart of every PACS is a hierarchical database into which details of all image files stored are populated and indexed (in the form Patient > Study > Image for easy retrieval; **Fig. 4.2**).

Image Lifecycle Management

Historic film libraries had a team of clerks working to remove and recycle 'out-of-date' films (by sending for silver reclamation). Cardboard film packets of deceased patients or those without recent imaging were also completely destroyed to free up space. These tasks were completed using small stickers, which were folded over the spine of the cardboard envelopes to indicate the year of last image, or whether the patient was paediatric, under cancer pathways, or involved in litigation. Each of these had different 'retention rules', meaning that their destruction should only take place a predetermined number of years from this last date. These rules continue today in the formalised NHS Records Management Code of Practice, which consolidates various legislative requirements on retention as well as best practice guidance. In practice, however, while informatics professionals should be aware of them, these rules are rarely followed. Instead, almost all UK hospitals choose to maintain PACS and RIS records indefinitely, currently because very few PACS (or RIS) provide image lifecycle management owing to the complexity of applying the differing rules, and comparative low cost of storage versus the cost of manual human interventions and potential expenditure for litigation risks if just one critical image is deleted incorrectly. There is discussion whether this current practice of indefinite retention of radiology records breaches principle 5 of the Data Protection Act (DPA) 1998 (kept for longer than is required for the original purpose), or equivalent in the upcoming General Data Protection Regulation (GDPR), and places an obligation on PACS Managers to create lifecycle policies.

While it is currently common practice for all images to be retained indefinitely, this practice is expected to change in the 2020s owing to digital archives swelling in size, along with the partial adoption of vendor neutral archives (VNAs) of which the majority contain some form of lifecycle management (which can be based on similar non-clinical uses, such as the archival of email).

Deconstructed PACS and Open Source PACS

Deconstructed PACS are those where individual portions of the application have been selectively 'cut-away' from the whole package. These types of PACS are popular in some areas that have well-developed surrounding systems, such as EPRs with universal viewers, or for those sites who may ingest images but have no need to view them (perhaps private providers who acquire imaging but do not report in-house, rather their business is to send imaging on for viewing/reporting elsewhere, thereby not requiring a viewer or any kind of image processing capabilities).

Open Source PACS are an extension of the general principles of crowd development – whereby the source code (the written machine instructions to run the applications) are made freely available for anyone to edit and contribute to. The benefits of this approach are that development of features, patching of security issues, and the incorporation of new technologies is potentially rapid; however, this approach requires experienced developers familiar with the programming language used. Open Source PACS are currently popular in countries such as South Korea, China, and Malaysia because of their flexibility and low cost. A very low percentage of Open Source PACS is being used in the UK or other western countries because the various strict regulatory requirements are more difficult to meet with this approach. However, a team was formed within NHS Digital to explore the options around this, with a focus on cost saving.

VNA

A somewhat misleading term, VNAs are archives intended to serve multiple applications (perhaps ingesting images from radiology, cardiology, and pathology PACS plus even wider non-medical applications) with a single universal viewer to unify the presentation of data. A shared patient identifier is crucial to their operation. VNAs are actually provided and maintained by a vendor, typically in a proprietary manner, albeit usually separate from any of the PACS application suppliers. In the mid-2010s, these storage systems were heavily promoted by well-funded non-medical IT software marketing departments as being a solution to enterprise-wide storage and access to images acquired across multiple departments. Although beneficial on paper, in many cases organisations that did install VNAs remain using their functionality purely as if they were simple PACS storage archives, neglecting the additional features that would deliver value on the investment of these more expensive archives. VNAs were also marketed as allowing for easier migration between PACS suppliers (with simply disconnecting the outgoing archive and connecting the incoming archive being necessary); however, there remains the more complex consideration of migrating between VNA suppliers when these are changed themselves.

There are five established levels of VNA:

- *Level 1:* the equivalent of a standard historic PACS archive (all images saved in DICOM format and identified by accession numbers).
- *Level 2:* the equivalent of a modern PACS archive (images can be saved and viewed in other formats, such as Joint Photographic Experts Group [JPEG] and audio video interleaved [AVI], but remain identified by accession numbers), which can be provided by multiple clinical information systems.

- *Level 3:* the equivalent of a multi-media archive with an almost universal acceptance of multi-media file formats, including portable document formats (.pdfs) and common report text formats.
- *Level 4:* builds on Level 3, with accessibility (storage and viewing capabilities) to several neighbouring sites.
- *Level 5:* stores any digital file, with full interoperability for sharing (rather than duplicating) data across multiple hospitals, regions, and even national boundaries.

Supplier Neutral Archives

A supplier neutral archive (SNA) is almost identical in functionality to VNAs but does not utilise the proprietary VNA supplier software for management of data. SNAs start life as a storage array provided by major suppliers, such as Dell, Hewlett Packard, or EMC, and rely on either Open-Source or 'homebrew' file management software to carry out the necessary functions.

Enterprise Archives

When marketed separately, enterprise archives (EAs) are typically SNAs with equivalent functionality to a Level 4 or Level 5 VNA. They represent the ultimate in supplier detachment and freedom, but require experienced staff to install, maintain, and manage them. EAs will almost exclusively rely on Open Source or locally maintained software to operate.

Image Viewing

Software to allow the viewing and manipulation of images is provided by all major PACS vendors at varying cost and functionality. Historically, a proprietary application was required to be installed by a system administrator on each workstation to be used for viewing, limiting the reach of PACS to those PCs themselves; modern systems now utilise functionality similar to that offered by 'Microsoft ClickOnce', allowing users unlimited installs. Zero-footprint viewers are now also available, so called because of their use of common web-based standards requiring no installation, no specialist plug-ins, or little beyond a supported web browser.

Progressing from this, in recent years great emphasis has been placed upon allowing 24/7 access to diagnostics. To facilitate this, remote viewing applications allow for the secure and reliable viewing of radiological images beyond the traditional boundaries of PACS without requiring network interconnections, such as VPNs, to be established. Offerings vary with software supplier, but with cloud-based PACS now no longer requiring on-premises storage, off-premises viewing is technologically possible and being developed by several of the major PACS vendors. Areas where this will provide great benefits include radiologist reviews at home or off-site night reporting facilities.

Importing and Exporting Images to a PACS

Importing

By far the most encountered method of importing images to a PACS is by the action of submitting an image or set of images from an image acquisition station. Other methods are directly via removable media (CD, DVD, Blu-Ray, portable hard drive), scanned via a digitiser, uploaded from files, such as those received by email, or via data sharing methods, such as the IEP. As an image or set of images is imported into a PACS, the system will analyse the files, create a folder for storage, and generate the necessary hierarchical database entries to allow for future access. This process can take several minutes.

Exporting

Moving images out of the PACS, perhaps for continuing care elsewhere, can be carried out either by copying images to removable media CD/DVD/Blu-Ray/USB), printing to thermal film or plain paper, or sending via teleradiology systems or one of a number of electronic data sharing systems. Reasons for exporting are covered in more detail in Chapter 10. It must be noted that when choosing an electronic data sharing solution, data must not be transferred outside of the European Union (EU) borders without adequate protection (this includes the 'transfer' to storage servers in the USA or other non-EU countries) in order to comply with the current DPA and GDPR.

Encryption of removable media. Although local hospital policies may be stricter, within the UK as a whole it has long been held that encryption of removable media is unnecessary when that removable media holds four or fewer patients and is conveyed to its destination in a secure manner (defined as either being with clinical notes using a specialist courier, or via a trackable delivery method).

Differences Between Departmental PACS

While based on similar technologies and backgrounds, cardiology and pathology PACS systems (as with their departmental workflows) have several inherent differences to radiology's, which make them slightly different to manage. These differences are set out in *Table 4.1.*

Table 4.1 Comparison of radiology, cardiology, and pathology PACS

Features	Radiology PACS	Cardiology PACS	Pathology PACS
Presentation	Single images in stacks if necessary	Videos	Single images
Average image/series size	Small (current average size similar to a high resolution photograph)	Large (current average similar to a low resolution video)	Very large (extremely high resolution HD images)
Average number of images per study	Many	Several	Under 20
Commonest format	DICOM	AVI	Currently lacking unified standardisation between vendors: proprietary TIF, SVS, CZI, NDPI, JPEG(/2000), WSI etc.

AVI, audio video interleaved; DICOM, digital imaging and communications in medicine; HD, high definition; JPEG, joint photographic experts group; PACS, picture archiving and communication system; TIF, tagged image file (format); WSI, whole slide image.

As a result of this, some hospitals choose to have each of the systems above managed by different specialist teams, with an overall Systems Manager co-ordinating the approaches.

Housekeeping

Each part of the imaging informatics environment involves some degree of human interaction. As humans (and to a lesser extent machines) make errors, these need to be identified and corrected on a daily basis in order to ensure the datasets stored are as complete and current as possible.

Common Housekeeping Tasks

Housekeeping tasks vary between systems and different vendors, common tasks are described below.

Mismatching/failed verification/unspecified reunions. Matching up incorrectly identified images on the PACS with their correct details. When changing examination, request, or patient details for studies, it is standard practice that PACS themselves do not alter the actual images. Instead, the existing images are left with the original demographics/ details intact, with an entry being created in a 'ledger' to indicate to the system to replace the original details with the 'corrected' details upon each access. This has no real impact in standard use; however, when migrating to a future replacement PACS, the images revert to the original details unless the changes in the ledger are also incorporated during the migration process. This is a common risk for migrations, and a reason why some hospitals prefer to create frozen archives rather than risk scenarios where years of housekeeping efforts may be reversed.

Worklist maintenance. Reporting and clinical staff typically operate from worklists, which require regular review after service or equipment changes to ensure they remain current and are providing complete lists.

Empty exams and unreported study lists. Undertaking safety checks to identify where human or machine error has resulted in either images being placed in the wrong location, not sent from the acquisition station (resulting in 'empty' exams), or left unreported for a longer time than expected (missing from reporting worklists).

Managing disk space demands on servers. Digital imaging, particularly CT, MR, and XA modalities, are utilising an ever increasing amount of space per study. This task is simply making sure the system has enough space to continue operating, or that appropriate actions are taken.

Backups. Undertaking regular backups (daily in most cases) and verifying that the backups will actually work, if needed.

Artefact recognition and reject analysis. As with film-based radiography, artefacts in digital imaging have existed from the inception of the technology. Artefacts are specific to the modalities and equipment utilised and should be guarded against as much as practicable to avoid reducing the diagnostic accuracy of the imaging, or the need to repeat any radiation exposure. Informatics staff play a vital role in this, because they have routine oversight of multiple modalities. Reject analysis also provides an overview of the causes of re-irradiation throughout an institution, which can provide valuable insights into beneficial practice, technique, or equipment changes that are not visible to individual image acquisition practitioners.

Upgrade planning. In the short term, from the moment a PACS is installed, it begins to age. As a medical device, there is generally a lag of around 1 year or so between new features being developed by modality vendors and these being made available in new versions of PACS software (to allow for the development, testing, and regulatory validation cycle). As medicine is continually evolving as technology improves, a PACS needs regular upgrades, at least once a year to stay current and secure.

Over the longer term, when replacing an entire PACS, there is a choice: move all data to a new system completely through a period of migration or, alternatively, to create a separate frozen archive of the legacy data using either the existing hardware or new, modern hardware. While the convenience of having all data in one location is a primary consideration, the cost and risks of carrying this out may make it preferable in some cases to utilise the frozen archive process. The frozen archive process creates a clear separation between the old and the new systems and allows for any historic bad housekeeping (particularly around matching up incorrectly identified studies) not to 'contaminate' the new system – effectively a fresh start can be made. This combined with the anticipated failure of some images to be successfully migrated during a migration process (leading to them being abandoned), makes frozen archives appeal in practice more than on paper.

Facilitating CAB/CAGs. Held in larger sites, the Change Advisory Board (CAB) is a more formal version of the informal Change Advisory Group (CAG) process used in smaller sites. These regular meetings consist of a number of individuals representative of the users of the system, plus the System Managers. The group or board hears proposals for changes (e.g. introduction of new features or rearranging layouts) and votes upon them.

Incident investigations. Essentially working out what happened/went wrong in critical incidents as they are reported, this task involves researching the history of images and auditing their use to provide input into wider investigations.

CHAPTER 5

RIS, MPI AND OTHER TEXT SYSTEMS

While images are the most visible output from a Radiology department into the wider clinical environment, text-based systems also play a vital role. The most prevalent of these are covered in this chapter.

Radiology Information System

RIS is the generic name for an application or group of applications used to handle the textual data related to imaging procedures, such as examination details, attendance lists, appointment diaries, reports, and billing data. It also includes data required under the Ionising Radiation (Medical Exposure) Regulations (IR[ME]R) (e.g. radiation dose, referrer, and operator details) and Ionising Radiation Regulations (IRR) (radioisotope data), as well as the Medicines Act 1968 (any prescription-only pharmaceuticals administered as part of the imaging exam, such as contrast in IVU [intravenous urography] or glyceryl trinitrate in CT imaging). Predominantly a text-based application (with scanned paper forms being available also in many cases), the first RISs were simply created as a replacement to the paper diaries widely used at the time, necessary as workloads increased, the types of examinations offered broadened, and departments grew to the point where it was difficult to continue using a single book to track multiple rooms with widely differing appointment slot lengths.

From a technology perspective, just as with the imaging output from radiological examinations, the textual data generated within the department is also structured, and this lends itself to being placed within a tabular database structure, with individual components of an entry picked out and placed upon the screen in the correct places. However, as the vast majority of the data a RIS handles is text, the scale and size of the hardware required to operate the application is significantly smaller.

By their nature, RISs are unique to Radiology; other departments have similar systems tailored to their textual workflows, known generically as clinical information systems (CISs). For example, Pathology utilises a LIMS (laboratory information management system).

Looking to the future, some major software manufacturers have begun to incorporate the functionality of RISs into their other applications, as can be seen in *Table 5.1*.

Today, as so many functions of a traditional text-based RIS are being subsumed into other surrounding systems, it is becoming questionable whether in the future they will continue to exist as a separate application, with the removal of an interface bringing benefits to departments in the form of increases in reliability.

Key Terminology

Accession numbers. These are a unique identifier given to studies, usually allocated from the RIS within the Radiology department, sent via a worklist to the modality, and passed both from the RIS (to create a folder) and from the modality (as part of the images) to PACS for storage. Accession numbers are typically sequential and, in NHS sites, are in the majority of cases prefixed with the hospital's national site organisation data service identifier (ODS code) to help keep them nationally unique: a useful feature when sharing images.

Examination ID. The use of examination identification (ID) will vary depending on the RIS provider used. Many RIS suppliers utilise a sequential number given to each examination that forms part of the same attendance (e.g. an attendance may be booked with a left and right hand – two exams – each with the same accession number, but

Table 5.1 Modern distribution of traditional RIS functionality among other systems

Core functionality	Current use	Historic replacement of	Being replaced by
Reporting of radiological studies	Input and storage of reports (master index of reports)	Cardboard report slips	PACS-based reporting
Appointments	Booking/pending and storage of future appointments	Paper diaries	Scheduling functionality in EPR systems
Worklists	Generation of worklists for on-screen reference/ sending to image acquisition stations	Time ordered pile of request cards	EPR-originated worklists
Statistics	Provision of aggregated data to a body of the Department of Health (currently the Health and Social Care Information Centre) for payments and performance monitoring	Superintendent/ district radiographers' reports	Business data warehouse software run and managed at an enterprise level across multiple discrete systems to unify data collection into a single tool

EPR, electronic patient record; PACS, picture archiving and communication system; RIS, radiology information system.

with 01 and 02 as the examination ID). However some suppliers opt to use a permanently fixed examination ID of 0 or 00, preferring to vary the accession number in these cases instead. This lack of standardisation sometimes hampers reporting processes when shared between hospitals with different RIS providers.

NICIP. Initially, in order to allow for easier recording and reporting, a national examination code list was created. Known as the National Interim Clinical Imaging Procedure (NICIP) Code Set this encompasses all possible radiological examinations undertaken in the UK. This code set is used extensively across the country, and is, for example, the basis for the XCHES abbreviations entered in examination details for chest X-ray examinations. The prefix of the codes indicates the modality – X being 'plain film', C being CT, M being MRI, and so forth. Similar standardised lists exist for other departments.

The NICIP code set is proprietary data to the NHS, and requires a subscription to receive the regular updates.

SNOMED-CT. Aimed to eventually replace the NICIP codes, the Systematised Nomenclature Of Medicine – Clinical Terms (SNOMED-CT) is intended to be a pan-organisational standard health terminology list covering all clinical disciplines, and is essentially an internationally recognised vocabulary. It is currently not widely adopted within radiology, but has the potential to provide greater detail on procedures and interoperation with wider parts of a healthcare organisation's informatics environment (particularly with other systems, outside radiology). SNOMED-CT is a marketed product of the Heath Terminology Standards Development Organisation. Utilising SNOMED-CT will allow for greater detail to be recorded in forthcoming electronic healthcare records (EHRs), as better coding of data will allow for greater use of machine-based processing, including health prediction algorithms and automated follow-ups.

ODS (NACS). Another national code list, the ODS list [still commonly known by its former name of National Administrative Code Service (NACS)] provides a list of abbreviations to identify each healthcare provider within the UK. For example, these abbreviations take the form of RT3 (Royal Brompton and Harefield NHS Foundation Trust), RV8 (London North West Healthcare NHS Trust), and RTX (University Hospitals of Morecambe Bay NHS Foundation Trust), and should be used to prefix all generated accession numbers, local room identifiers, and imaging acquisition station AETs (see Chapter 8) to allow for easy identification by external sites (e.g. after a data transfer). Originally leaving imaging acquisition station names to the discretion of the installing engineer (resulting in hundreds of A&E Room 1s across the country!) was previous bad practice, which current PACS teams should work to resolve as stations are updated or replaced.

Master Patient Index

Falling under a variety of names depending on the software brand in place, the MPI is also commonly known as the HIS (hospital information system) or PAS (patient administration system). It is a database application, which primarily stores the demographic and contact details of patients, as well as any national identifiers (NHS, community health index [CHI: Scottish national identifier], Health & Care [H&C] number, etc.) and local identifiers (the 'Hospital Number'). As an MPI is designed to be the Master Index, demographic changes in this master database, including the addition of new patients, are passed down to almost every other imaging informatics and hospital system (an exception being maternity information systems, which require the ability to 'pass back up' the notification of a birth and consequently create a new MPI record for the new life). This 'cascade' update process ensures that the records on other systems each match the primary details recorded in the MPI. Communication between the MPI and other text-based imaging informatics components is usually carried out using the HL7 standard (Chapter 9). MPIs are one of the oldest hospital informatics applications, and frequently remain running on emulators of long since discontinued hardware (giving common systems the nickname 'green screen' in light of the formatting of green text on black background, reminiscent of the historic computer terminals available in libraries for database searching. The downward cascade of data can be seen in **Fig. 5.1**.

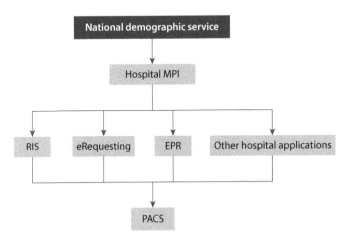

Fig. 5.1 Typical downward flow of demographic data originating from an MPI. (EPR, electronic patient record; MPI, master patient index; PACS, picture archiving and communication system; RIS, radiology information system.)

Electronic Patient Record

The EPR is a method of storing a patient's medical records and notes electronically rather than in bound paper bundles, which are difficult to search (and sometimes read). EPRs include a viewer application to allow for clinicians and other authorised healthcare staff (and in some instances the patient themselves) to read and add to the records, just as if they remained paper based. As digitising the billions of pages of historic paper medical notes will take time to accomplish and allow EPRs to become mainstream, it is anticipated that EPR applications will gradually move to include PACS images and RIS data over the coming years.

eRequesting

eRequesting systems (OCSs) allow referrers to place requests for a range of diagnostic tests (including radiology examinations) into a single online application, which then directly sends the request to the relevant department, removing the paper 'transit delay' and potential for loss/misdirection. These systems also offer a range of tracking functions to allow clinicians to view the status of their request, as well as the report when available. eRequesting is popular within healthcare institutions as it removes the need for a paper request form to be conveyed physically to a collection point, allows multiple people to view the request (lessening the chances of duplicate requests), and also provides higher quality audit data. Within the UK, Pathology departments were the initial adopters of eRequesting: primarily owing to the workflow in this department requiring a request to accompany the test (rather than the request being placed in advance, as for the bulk of radiology studies). Departments utilising eRequesting but choosing to print out the forms as they reach the correct area in the Radiology department for practitioners to use during the examination are said to be paper-lite.

Dose Management/Dose Monitoring Software

Numerous studies have examined whether the move from film- and chemical-based radiology to digital systems has increased doses, particularly in CR radiography examinations. Now, with dose information being recorded directly in RIS, dose analysis and management software is becoming popular to identify trends and provide feedback to radiographers who may be identified as having better (or worse) techniques than others. This software also allows the automated identification of ageing or failing equipment requiring service/replacement.

National Healthcare Numbers (National Patient Identifiers)

Historically, and in many cases still to this day, different healthcare institutions have utilised different local identifiers (Hospital Numbers) to record what could be the same patients. As there is no central database ensuring these local numbers are not repeated elsewhere (and thus potentially they could be identifying different patients in different parts of the country), hazards were identified at the turn of the millennium. Given that sharing and cross-organisational working is now so much more likely, safe image transfers and interorganisational working depend on a common shared national healthcare identifier. Indeed, regional EHR systems now depend on having a single 'master' identifier per patient record across multiple healthcare sites. This is sometimes one of the most difficult aspects to begin setting up, as despite the multitude of other identifiers already being in existence in countries, healthcare records may require to be kept separate from other governmental functions (taxation, housing, voter registration, etc.) for increased privacy purposes. Even within the UK, national healthcare numbers vary depending on the systems in use in the respective regions. For example, England, Wales, and the Isle of Man utilise the NHS Number (a sequential 9 digit number from an allowable range with a final 10th check-digit calculated by a modulus 11 mathematical operation for input error checking); Scotland chooses the CHI Number (created by the patient's date of birth in format DDMMYY, 3 sequential digits with one transposed to indicate gender, with the same final check-digit as for England) and Northern Ireland the H&C Number (sequential, as in England). All three of these national numbers are rendered in 3-3-4 number format and have agreed ranges such that numbering will not overlap. Somewhat inefficiently, when travelling between the different regions, fresh numbers are allocated in the new regions to supplement the existing numbers. This could mean that despite a patient being able to move freely between England and Scotland for treatment, they may well hold two different electronic health records for themselves if no link is created between the 'master' national numbers. The NHS Spine Demographics Application holds the national database of NHS numbers for England, and similar smaller systems exist for other countries. The formatting of the various national identifiers in use within the UK is illustrated in **Fig. 5.2**.

Many other countries have also long adopted national healthcare identifiers, such as Australia (Individual Healthcare Identifier – IHI), New Zealand (National Health Index – NHI Number), and Canada (Universal Person Identifier/Client Registry). Yet more have simply cross-purposed existing systems for healthcare, such as those originally for taxation: the Personal Identity Number in Sweden being a prime

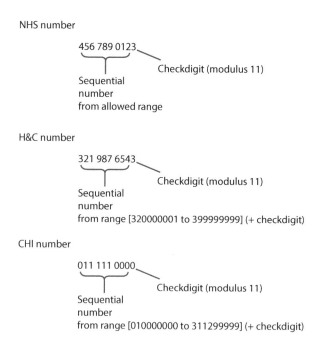

Fig. 5.2 UK national health identifiers. (CHI, community health index; H&C, health and care; NHS, National Health Service.)

example (originally a tax identifier, but now somewhat astonishingly far more widely utilised and readily quoted by residents than UK identifiers in many different situations).

Denmark, Norway, and Finland also utilise a similar system to Scotland incorporating demographics into the number, primarily for age-related screening, benefit, and gender service segregation.

Other countries looking to reduce duplication and paper usage in healthcare settings are also beginning to introduce single healthcare identifiers. For example, in the Republic of Ireland, a national healthcare identifier has very recently (autumn 2016) been brought into service, shortly also after the introduction of postcodes (Eircodes) in summer 2015 as another national database.

Discussion over which healthcare system has created the 'best' national healthcare identifier is long considered by other countries wishing to introduce similar schemes. It is notable that the English and Northern Irish systems allow for user anonymity, as no demographics are encoded in the number, whereas other countries with demographics allow for easier recognition and inclusion of specific health initiatives. With international migration and even travel for healthcare reasons now becoming commonplace, determining an international healthcare identifier will soon be a consideration. Currently, the closest available to a global identifier is the passport MRZ (machine readable zone: the alphanumeric line at the bottom of the passport photo page), which is intended to be globally unique. Unfortunately, many individuals around the world do not have passports (USA statistics show only around one-third of American residents holds a passport) and some individuals hold two or more (in a similar manner to some individuals holding two or more NHS numbers despite the intention not to).

Wider NHS Services

eReferral Service (formerly branded as NHS Choose & Book)

In England, patients have long had the choice to choose their own preferred NHS healthcare provider rather than being assigned to their GP or consultant's choice. A self-service online booking service originally provided a choice of the closest four or five treatment centres, but now offers a wider choice. Some radiology services are moving to integrate with this system, removing the burden on appointments clerks making telephone calls and posting letters as patients begin to manage their own journey through the diagnostic process.

NBSS/NBSP

The National Breast Screening Service (NBSS) is effectively a Hitachi RIS tailored to the National Breast Screening Programme to co-ordinate and run clinics. A similar system (NBSP) is run in the Republic of Ireland by IBM. NBSS/NBSP patients have their own identifiers for this service, resulting in additional processes being required by PACS teams to match records if the patient attends multiple services. NBSS and NBSP integrate into PACS in the same manner as conventional RISs.

CHAPTER 6

INTEGRATING WITH OTHER SYSTEMS

- Imaging informatics does not exist in the healthcare environment in a vacuum.
- Examining the wider healthcare system environment outside radiology shows a growing trend for systems to interconnect and exchange data.
- As a frequently unknown and complex area, understanding the drivers behind integration and considering potential futures will arm those interested in imaging informatics to be prepared as technology evolves.

Large volumes of digital data are generated in a healthcare environment, with imaging departments being just one contributor. Owing to the now routine use of intradepartmental CISs, all radiographers, laboratory practitioners, physiotherapists and many other allied health professionals (AHP) are involved on a daily basis with the uses and applications of the field of health informatics. In some cases, these CISs are already integrated, allowing vital healthcare data to complement that already recorded in one speciality. Having this interaction with each other allows for an easier multidisciplinary approach to healthcare, and encourages discrete departments, such as Imaging, to contribute to a patient's 'cradle to the grave' dataset, which ultimately will become their EHR. As a result of this, it is apt that interconnections serve a large portion of the current work that a modern imaging informatics professional undertakes. While the examples given in this chapter are on diagnostic imaging, the concepts can be applied to the laboratory information systems that are following similar flows, albeit with practitioners having differing levels of physical patient contact.

Interoperability is the capacity of two or more systems to share and communicate, allowing collaboration within an organisation or between other 'businesses'/people/IT systems, of which there are various levels.

Towards the Interoperability of Clinical Information Systems: A History

1950s

The concept of using computers in healthcare was introduced in the 1950s for billing and finance reasons (at the time, computers were extremely large, extremely expensive, and required specialist technical skills to operate, limiting their further usefulness).

1960s and 70s

In the following decades, PAS began to be developed in the UK to store a patient's demographic information (commonly name, address, contact details, date of birth, and unique patient ID). The most recognisable widely used early 'clinical' system was the IRC PAS (initially run by the company ICL, then Siemens Nixdorf), which came to popularity in the UK during these years. Related development of clinically related systems also began, primarily to reduce the paper 'diaries' and 'address books' that were beginning to become cumbersome in individual departments across the healthcare enterprise.

1980s and 90s

During this era, CIS became commonplace, and more activity related to attendances began to be recorded. However, the various systems in place did not widely communicate with each other. To create records on a CIS using details from a PAS at the time involved staff looking on one system then transcribing the information over to another manually, meaning the data may not have been necessarily identical (or correct) because of the possibility of human error creeping in during the manual transfer process (or even possibly because the data were incomplete in the first place).

As a result of this inefficiency, there were many drivers to ensure both the hospital-wide and CISs integrated with each other to assist in the management of relevant data, and to help with the efficiency of healthcare workers, thereby improving the quality of patient care. From this period until the millennium, clinical systems were evolving for all the healthcare specialities to various degrees, from 'the therapies' having administrative and document management type systems for scheduling and patient administration, to diagnostic systems building on the administrative aspects and having clinical information flows requiring inputs from the departmental patient/sample journeys, not just entries at the beginning and end of the patient experience for the relevant department. It was also hoped to reduce paper so that information was shared electronically rather than on hardcopies, which could be lost or changed without the information system being updated. These requirements resulted in suppliers developing their CISs so that they could interact with associated systems, such as imaging modalities and laboratory equipment. Once images/laboratory results were being captured electronically, ways of sharing the information were developed to allow images as well as textual imaging reports, attendance details, and so on, to be stored and shared in a readable format (where they were usually then printed on paper and film). This would fulfil a patient's expectations that their records should be held digitally and shared when needed.

2000s and 2010s

CISs were by now used in many individual departments, with demographic feeds being provided by local and ultimately national MPIs. The modern streamlined MPI of demographics utilises more recent developments in technology and programming to allow more rapid searches together with selective querying plus connectivity to research, epidemiological, planning, and statistical systems or databases as required.

Emerging from the IRC PAS-era, these MPIs form the backbone of healthcare demographics distribution. Owing to the continued goal of paper-lite/paperless working, there has also been a natural move towards an EHR; diagnostic services began to contribute to this by sharing the information being stored on the relevant local CIS, usually as copies of the textual reports and sometimes alongside associated images.

Data from CISs are now being captured for numerous reasons, including activity, billing, or for national statistics, and these data are being copied into data warehouses that can be interrogated to avoid the possibility of impacting on performance of the live system if a large report is run.

Currently, the focus is moving towards providing functionality focussing on the needs of the patient, including giving the patients the information they need rather than storing it within the walls of the institution that obtained it.

In order to understand the process required for integration, the systems commonly available within organisations are described below and in **Fig. 6.1,** showing their position within an enterprise.

- *Strategic and administrative:*
    - Social media: messaging and other communication platforms.
    - Business intelligence (which consumes and processes the data generated by all these systems below to produce information required).
- *Administrative and operational:*
    - Enterprise resource planning facilitates the organisation-wide integration of complex processes and functions rather than relying on stand-alone systems.
    - Document management systems holding scanned and other documents in a relatively structured and searchable manner.
- *Operational and clinical:*
    - Enterprise-wide systems, such as EHR, document management systems, PACS, MPI.
    - CISs, such as LIMS, RIS.
- *Clinical and strategic:*
    - Computerised physician order entry (eRequesting).
    - Internal portals.
    - Patient personal healthcare record (PHR).

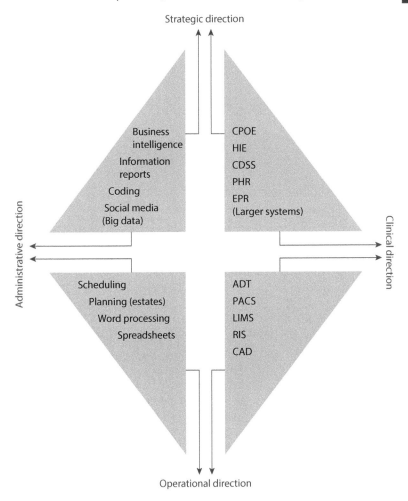

Fig. 6.1 Systems commonly available and their direction and overlap. *Note:* not all these systems are integrated, some stand alone. (ADT, admit, discharge, or transfer; CAD, computer aided diagnosis; CDSS, clinical decision support system; CPOE, computerised physician order entry; EPR, electronic patient record; HIE, health information exchange; LIMS, laboratory information management system; PACS, picture archiving and communication system; PHR, personal health record; RIS, radiology information system.)

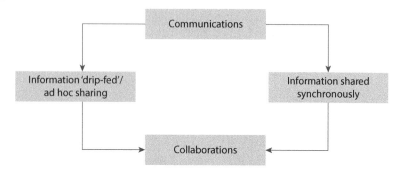

Fig. 6.2 Collaborations and communications.

These four types of systems encourage electronic interoperability, reducing the need for hard copies of patient data to pass between departments, thereby promoting simpler collaboration.

As shown in **Fig. 6.2**, collaboration itself builds upon the capabilities of the communications infrastructure, whether this is performed asynchronously (each direction at different times) or, more preferably, synchronously (both communicating at the same time) and is frequently the main focus for achieving agreed specific targets/objectives for improving patient care in an organisation, such as results being available to all healthcare staff that need them.

When future gazing, it is expected that by 2025 these systems will be interacting with patients, giving them electronic access/management to their EHR, with the prospect of decision support systems in place to intervene if required. The concepts of the approach below can also be used for therapy (radiotherapy) and other diagnostic departments, such as laboratory information systems in Pathology, owing to the common information flows around integration and interoperability being applicable to all.

Achieving Interoperability

There are currently a number of ways that systems can interact to achieve interoperability, which have been split into two areas. First, an understanding of the technical aspects of the systems is needed to ensure the information is delivered correctly. Second, we need to ensure that the theoretical processes are understood (and in place) in order that the various systems can understand the relevant information, the latter being the most difficult. The introduction of new technologies will not automatically resolve a badly organised department, and sometimes this can uncover deeper deficiencies within the organisations, resulting in a greater focus being on the 'business' (in this sense, the way processes are followed) rather than the software.

Infrastructure Decisions/Options

The infrastructure that both current and future systems will be run upon needs to be considered by the whole organisation; possible architecture that may already be in place or being driven towards, with diagnostics able to collaborate and influence the decisions are shown in **Fig. 6.3.**

- *Limited integration between a few systems (minimum integration):*
  - Imaging and limited 'sharing' systems, i.e. a system that has little interaction with other systems (MPI/PACS/RIS).
  - The MPI/PACS and RIS along with an archive (commonly historically known as a VNA, despite being provided and supported by a vendor itself).
- *Integration within the organisation (medium integration):*
  - Imaging (MPI/PACS/RIS + archive) along with OCS (via HL7 messaging), which allows for interoperability between other systems.
  - Imaging (MPI/PACS/RIS/OCS + archive) and decision support systems adding Laboratory/Pharmacy/Scheduling/Wards (including Emergency departments) and Therapy, again with HL7 messaging.
- *Integration with external organisations (high level of integration):*
  - Addition of health information exchanges (HIE)/primary community/mental plus sexual health services/portals for patients and clinicians.
  - With the merger of some organisations there may be two or three different CISs (RIS), which will still need to communicate with each other until a single instance (one larger merged system) is procured later.

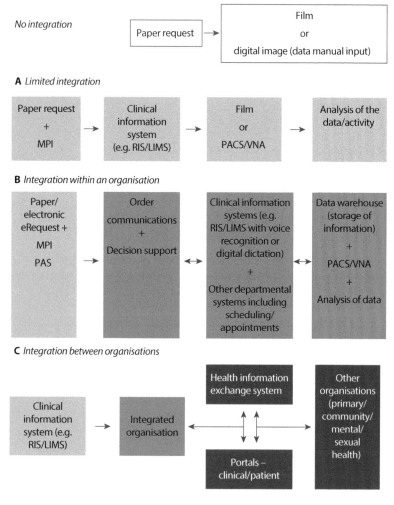

Fig. 6.3 Infrastructure options. (MPI, master patient index; PACS/VNA, picture archiving and communication system/vendor neutral archive; RIS/LIMS, radiology information system/laboratory information management system.)

In order to achieve any of these infrastructure options, there are several options:

Single system encompassing all. One supplier providing the majority of the components (from MPI to RIS) individually (or as a single system) would result in seamless communications, simply because the data will be stored on fewer databases (perhaps even just one). There are a number of Radiology PACS suppliers who integrate RIS into the PACS (making RIS + PACS a single application), but this is not commonplace in the UK.

Point-to-point model. As shown in **Fig. 6.4,** this is where multiple systems have **direct** connections to each other and thus have no single point of failure, which could also occur with the single system (the individual components, such as RIS/PACS or LIMS, can continue to operate if other sections of the system are unavailable). This method requires multiple connections with increasing complexity, as although two systems would require just one connection, five systems would require 10 connections and 10 systems would require 45 and so on, which is increasingly difficult to maintain with less centralised activity monitoring possible.

Hub and spoke model. This model (**Fig. 6.5**) reduces the number of connections as an integration engine (commonly known in the UK as a hub or broker) links the various systems, reducing the need to maintain each connection as for the point-to-point model. This can be managed by a central hub, and has the advantages of being able to choose the CIS needed (not reliant on one supplier providing all), with the main point of failure becoming the actual integration engine. Currently it appears that organisations are naturally following this model, especially when they have systems in place that need replacing at different times because of financial or support limitations.

In choosing the optimum model, there are tools to enable one to make an informed decision, such as the 2015 *Interoperability Handbook*, in which there is an 'interoperability decision tree' and detailed explanations of the various options.

Three connections between three systems

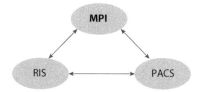

Ten connections to maintain between five systems

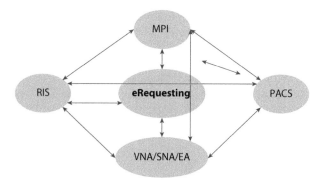

Forty-five connections to maintain between 10 systems (only one system's connections demonstrated), 36 more connections needed:

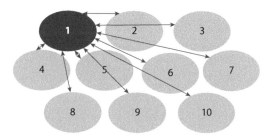

Fig. 6.4 The point-to-point model. (EA, enterprise archive; MPI, master patient index; PACS, picture archiving and communication system; RIS, radiology information system; SNA, supplier neutral archive; VNA, vendor neutral archive.)

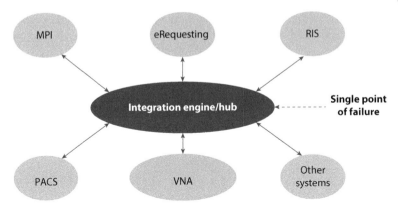

Fig. 6.5 The hub and spoke model. (MPI, master patient index; PACS, picture archiving and communication system; RIS, radiology information system; VNA, vendor neutral archive.)

Key Building Blocks of Interoperability

Patient ID

To make interoperability truly work throughout the systems, the patient will need a single patient identifier (an item in common with other systems) that is available to all organisations in order to support collaborative working. If there is not a common identifier, another option is the use of regional numbers, but this results in a confusing number of multiple identifiers.

Open Application Program Interfaces

There is an expectation that suppliers will need to work together more in the future to enable systems to be more interoperable; supplying an open and fully documented application program interface (API) that conforms to existing guidance assists this process. This will allow the relevant information to be made available, thereby reducing supplier lock-in and encouraging software house development teams to work together.

Best Practice

Interoperability following the actual deployment of CISs has proven difficult; e.g. in Denmark there has been a shift in the state-led hospitals with EPR systems from sharing data between themselves to regional collaborations, brought about because of changes in organisational responsibilities (Kierkegaard, 2015). Following the achievement of interoperability, benefits began to be realised, such as the flow of meaningful data (for the clinical and administrative processes), the ability to redesign processes, monitor quality (including patient safety), and being able to retrieve data from frozen legacy systems, as required.

Current Flows (with Limited Interoperability)

For an organisation with basic informatics infrastructure (solely PACS and RIS for radiology), the generic diagnostic information flows as part of a standard patient attendance can be categorised as below:

1　Initial patient interactions.
2　Clinician and patient interactions.
3　Diagnostic interactions.
4　Results.
5　Results distribution and further collaborative steps (**Fig. 6.6**).

Current Common Information Flows for Patients Needing Diagnostics

1 Initial Patient Interactions

- 1A Patient (or carer) identifies need to consult a healthcare professional.

2 Clinician and Patient Interactions

- 2A Patient presents to healthcare professional after having details taken, appointment arranged on a system or walking into a clinic/centre where details are entered into the relevant local system.
- 2B Patient examined and consultation recorded in local (unshared) system.
- 2C Patient referred for diagnostics (paper request form or eRequest).

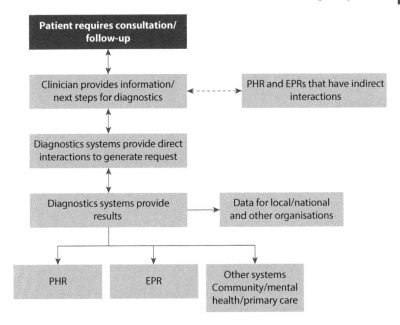

Fig. 6.6 eResult distribution/further collaborative steps. (EPR, electronic patient record; PHR, personal health record.)

3 Diagnostic Interactions

- 3A Request arrives at diagnostics department (with sample if laboratory).
- 3B Patient request interrogated/vetted by diagnostics department and entered onto the CIS.
- 3C Patient either scheduled for an appointment or the examination/test is performed immediately (skip to 3H if performed immediately).
- 3D If a patient has an appointment scheduled, a notification will either be presented to them immediately or sent later via another format (e.g. SMS/telephone/email/post).
- 3E Patient arrives for examination/test.
- 3F Examination/test information shared with imaging/laboratory modalities.
- 3G Examination/test performed/processed on relevant modality.

- 3H Data from examination/test sent for interpreting and records made on the relevant CIS (RIS and PACS for radiology, LIMS for pathology).
- 3I Patient will be discharged from diagnostic department.

4 Results

- 4A Results, if interpreted, will be sent to the referrer or teams.
- 4B Results will also be available locally, within the healthcare organisation.
- 4C Data can be sent, or summary reports run, for internal or external parties.

5 Results Distribution and Further Collaborative Steps

- 5A Data may be shared via proprietary systems if required to further the patient's treatment at another institution.

Changes to interoperability are fairly common as new technologies and uses of data arise. Current information flows need to be documented (*steps 1A–5A above*), typically via a flow diagram, prior to any changes to ensure that the future flows do not mistakenly remove any of the critical components that will make it more difficult for the relevant teams and the patient. These concepts can be modified and also for other services similar to diagnostics, such as cardiology, surgery, and electronic prescription services (sending prescriptions to a choice of pharmacies).

Conceptual Future Interoperability Flows

The future flows over the next decade are expected to follow similar concepts but with increasing levels of technology involved. There initially appear to be more steps to the future information flows (below) than the current flows (above); however, these could save resources, such as time and costs, and may not need inputs/user interventions as systems become more highly interoperable. Some of the future flows may already be performed to certain degrees as, over the life of this book, different organisations will be progressing more quickly than others. There is also an increasing emphasis on the use of integrating the healthcare enterprise (IHE) profiles and a push for organisational systems that already communicate with each other via an EPR to be able to do so bi-directionally (e.g. in radiology PACS-based reporting requires a two-way link to RIS).

1 Patient Only Interaction (Initial)

1A Patient interacts with the health service provider via a PHR that they can manage, starting their journey leading to diagnostics. For this to occur it is crucial that there is what is known as 'semantic interoperability' (each system can understand the different types and formatting of information exchanged). To achieve this, SNOMED-CT exists and should be used. This semantic interoperability can be bi-directional (in both directions) and have the ability to link into more than one CIS. The patient's PHR may be tied to a single health provider (NHS Trust) but in the future will be positioned between several organisations, such as:

- Hospitals/clinics (medical/non-medical).
- GPs.
- Non-acute settings, such as community/mental and sexual health services.
- Private healthcare providers.
- Decentralised databases (research, statistics, etc.).

Research in 2016 showed that the underlying 'BlockChain' technology from the 'Bitcoin' project could be a useful way to secure PHRs when they may be updated by multiple organisations (the updates being stored in a verifiable 'chain' permanently). Studies have also found that there is an increasing appetite for patients to access their PHRs via social media if logistical and ethical issues were addressed. For patients themselves, this would certainly be the quickest way to access and manage health records (particularly for those with chronic conditions). Some countries have already introduced a 'light PHR' that patients can access and share, which will also link to services of relevant organisations. However, on the other hand, many nations are concentrating their efforts on increasing security and governance around health records making it, if anything, harder for patients to access their own records outside the walls of a hospital. This has so far raised a question: if patients/members of the public are able to access their financial records and share transactions between banks, then why not health records with healthcare organisations?

1B The patient uses a clinical decision support system (CDS) that has access to their records; data from certified devices can update the CDS with data for blood pressure and other vital signs, remotely and synchronously (with the potential for instant updates to the system maintaining them). Clinicians currently have access to electronic tools such iRefer (a resource previously known as 'Making the Best Use of a Radiology Department'), or sets of protocols that may be converted into an electronic decision tree, or a CDS. This CDS has the potential to be made patient accessible and friendly via a web-based application, driving patients towards it rather than less evidence-based tools, such as an internet search engine, or Wikipedia.

Wearable healthcare devices can support the synchronous updating of patient-provided measurement data by using relatively low cost mobile phone applications and wifi. The patient could also share their own information or comments by free text if necessary, including links to where their search engine had led them while they were trying to self-diagnose. For radiology, this information could be vital towards providing a clearer, more accurate patient history from contemporary notes at the time of the event occurrence, rather than relying on recall during consultation, dictation to a referrer, transcription, and compression onto a radiological request.

1C The CDS presents findings to the patient stating the options for access to a healthcare professional or is referred to another relevant pathway. These findings and recommendations from the CDS can be performed instantaneously, producing a link to the next step and also ensuring patient context is maintained (i.e. the patient not being required to re-enter their details for the next, albeit different, system). This will ensure a seamless experience for the user and also reduce the risk of the two systems not communicating, saving the patient time.

1D CDS or similar tool may directly arrange an appointment (if required). As the evidence-based protocols have been followed, both the patient and clinician will save time if a direct referral is made. This can also allow a selection of appointment times for the patient, reducing the risk of 'did-not-attend' (DNA).

1E If any preliminary diagnostics/information/preparation or any other reminders are needed, the patient will be prompted before the appointment. This is a simple computing query: <If> "(requirement for oral preparation)" occurs <Then> "(preparation delivered to patient or asked to collect it)" happens. This in turn will produce the information after the CDS has accessed the relevant data. This concept can be captured as an IHE mobile alert communications management (MACM) profile, sending alerts to patients/carers and also recording the outcomes on receipt of the alert.

1F The consultation, if needed, may be set up either face to face or via a unified communications system, which under the same platform may include video/audio calls, instant messaging, presence status, screen sharing capabilities, call control capabilities, voice recognition, and other methods of communication. An appointment system similar to those that are currently utilised may be used to schedule the initial consultation. Links will be found within the appointment to generate a unified communications session, or a face to face appointment if necessary or if this is preferred by the patient. The patient's choice is dependent on the waiting times or perceived convenience plus other preferences or needs. As well as the increasingly popular phone calls between patients and clinical practitioners for 'filtering' purposes (particularly for initial GP appointments), unified communication systems are available via various devices (desktops to mobile), which will allow communications via voice to video plus with the facility to share information digitally on a screen or by transferring data via the same platform. This allows the users to switch from video to screen sharing and provide flexibility for patient and healthcare staff to communicate with each other.

2 Clinician and Patient Interactions

2A At the consultation, the full EHR will be available along with results from the CDS (1C). At the time of the appointment the consultation will be either face to face or via unified communications with relevant documents/records shared with other health organisations using an IHE profile, such as cross-enterprise document sharing (XDS), allowing for rapid access to all relevant prior information.

2B With the patient's consent, all this can be recorded and added to their EHR for completeness. An IHE profile for this basic patient privacy consent (BPPC) is already available. Anecdotal reports from current practice show there are two schools of thought currently in use surrounding this: one being very strict and cautious around this type of record, and an opposing view promoting sharing as a way of increasing knowledge around a patient's choice and condition.

2C If Diagnostics are needed, the clinician's system will be able to interrogate the local healthcare organisation RIS/LIMS or EPR to determine where the patient may be sent via an eReferral or an eRequest, similar to choice exhibited via the PHR. Real-time waits and turnaround times can be calculated from the information held on RIS/LIMS appointment schedules, or via access to a local data warehouse where this information is normally copied (overnight or at the end of the working day). In the future, along with the real-time data, the initial costs of the diagnostics will be available along with pertinent information saving multiple telephone calls to various departments in a hospital. This ability to route requests to specific sites will present eRequesters with options to select a department based on an informed decision about waiting times, costs, or quality of service.

2D Subsequent to the location of the diagnostics being determined, the clinician's system will then communicate with the relevant system, such as the RIS/LIMS (if not already part of an EPR), by requesting the examination/test. There are order OCS or computerised physician order entry (CPOE) in place whereby eRequests ('orders' if laboratory/pharmacy related) are communicated and recorded in the relevant CIS. Updates will be bi-directional (from the CIS and the referring clinician's system) also reflecting the numerous statuses of the requests based on the request stages below (currently used interchangeably between imaging and pathology).

The sequential stages of a request (Radiology or other departments) are:

1 Requested.
2 Justified.
3 On hold (with reason).
4 Scheduled/booked.
5 Rescheduled (with reason).

6 DNA (with reason).
7 Started (examination).
8 Completed (examination).
9 Dictated.
10 Preliminary report.
11 Final report.
12 Addendum report.
13 Acknowledgment/report viewed.

There would be more information attached to each status to produce an audit trail, and create future information reports if required. This stage allows requests to be tracked much more easily, providing a transparent process for the patient and requestor.

The messages are sent using the current HL7 v2 standard for sending clinical and administrative data between software systems. However HL7 Fast Healthcare Interoperability Resources (FHIR) is a standalone exchange standard, which is starting to be considered as a communication standard for interoperability projects, as software authors understand interoperability is now a commercial selling point for their applications.

3 Diagnostic Interactions

3A Electronic referral/request arrives at diagnostics department (LIMS/RIS) with relevant data for patient (or with sample if laboratory). The eRequesting of imaging and other diagnostics is available from various software suppliers and this, despite the differing user interfaces, involves standard HL7 messaging that can be accepted by the RIS/LIMS and the ability for status updates to be communicated to additional systems as necessary, particularly if the patient has to be seen by multiple clinical teams, so that they can see updates in their own CISs. Another option is to build on any eReferral systems, which are in place worldwide, by utilising the IHE profile for CDS/order appropriate tracking (CDS/OAT), which is based on the data entered, checking for the appropriateness of the request with alternatives suggested where appropriate.

3B If the referral/request fits relevant criteria and there are no contraindications or queries from the diagnostic department, this can be authorised for examination as long as relevant standard operating procedures (SOP) and protocols are adhered to. There are standard flows for the initial diagnostic flows, such as the IHE scheduled workflow, incorporating requesting the imaging, to acquisition, storage, and viewing.

3C If the request needs to be vetted/protocol-checked there should be adequate information on the request supported by any other seamless links to supplementary information. Information, such as previous images or reports, may be retrieved either internally or externally using the IHE cross-community access (XCA) for imaging (XCA-I) profile, which should support the vetting process, and the sharing of laboratory reports (XD-LAB). There may be a move to optimised image protocols when vetting, whereby each examination is tailored to the specific patient (Chang, 2008). This personalised service could add value to the imaging results, but could potentially be open to abuse for financial gain by those that vet the request and who will also perform and be paid for it (by choosing the combination of parameters triggering an examination of maximum 'value' to the provider to be requested).

3D If the patient is not examined immediately, an appointment date/time for diagnostics will either be presented immediately or sent to the patient if there were any queries that had to be resolved. Conceptually a diagnostic appointment is similar to the commonly occurring O/P appointment, i.e. referral communication received (request) that is then scheduled into the system according to speciality (modality). Hence some EPRs generate these imaging appointments from the same EPR system as the rest of the hospital. This could in effect allow the appointment system to be managed by a non-imaging department (O/P), as long as the relevant imaging protocols and SOPs were shared. In coming years it is predicted that EPR will take over the current RIS functionality for scheduling appointments, owing to the ability to co-ordinate multiple department attendances rather than just for Imaging (as RIS currently does, requiring frequent discussions/amendments if the patient has multiple clinic attendances on one day already).

3E Patient arrives for examination/test and checks themselves into the imaging department from home or at the department, using self check-in services. This is similar to the online check-in experience at airports where a user can confirm an appointment electronically. If they fail to do so within a certain period of time their appointment is given to another patient to reduce waiting times and achieve capacity (possibly allowing an I/P who is waiting for such a vacancy to arise to attend in their place). If a patient DNA, this will be recorded and sanctions, if relevant, may be imposed. There is also the possibility of using geo-informatics, the information science of geography to monitor persistent offenders (e.g. by requiring patients to have an application on a mobile device that can alert the hospital of the likelihood of a DNA by patient location, similar to tracking a taxi on an application that one may have requested online).

3F Examination/test information shared with imaging/laboratory modalities. The information that was first received in the original request (patient and exam details) will be enough to populate the relevant modalities, with supplementary information being entered by the radiographer, technician, or clerk if required. Owing to the interoperation of the various systems, the patient information will be consistent throughout, helping ensure patient safety on matters such as allergies or crucial medical information.

Before examining the patient they can be positively identified by using Quick Response (QR) or 3D bar codes either associated with the appointment letter, on a mobile device (or on a wristband if the patient in currently an I/P), or by a photographic record.

3G Patient status updates continuously on relevant real-time customisable dashboards displayed departmentally or for each modality. This is possible via RIS/PACS/EPR modules using dynamic worklists that will already be created to meet the user needs. These can be converted into a dashboard for staff (including those outside diagnostics, such as O/P departments waiting for their patients to return following a diagnostic test completion) and patients to see their real-time waits or queue position, similar to telephone on-hold wait time systems currently used for many companies.

3H Examination/test performed/processed on equipment. This modality will then produce a digital image (or result) that can be stored for interpretation. For radiology and pathology, the images should be of the well-established DICOM standard, which inherently allows easy sharing of the images to a suitable PACS or other archive.

3I Data from examination/test sent for interpreting and records made on the relevant CIS (RIS and PACS for radiology, LIMS for pathology). The results need to be sent and stored so that they can be interpreted easily in a variety of ways by specialist processing workstations or trained staff. New data that can be automatically added in the Radiology department is the dose information by utilising the IHE profile radiation exposure monitoring (REM).

Within Radiology, some departments may leave images unreported or classed as 'auto-reported' (approximately 47% of departments advised of this practice in a census issued by the Royal College of Radiologists in 2012). Hence there is a move towards identifying and training more advanced reporting practitioners to fill these gaps for reporting or utilising machine-based reporting (currently being developed by several companies, particularly for breast imaging in radiology and abnormal cell counts in pathology).

3J Patient will be 'discharged' from diagnostic department. Once the examination is completed and the patient is free to go, the scheduling information needs to be captured and closed, with notifications to interested parties, such as. referrers who wanted to view the images before a formal report was produced. This can be performed automatically once the examination is completed, with fields auto-populated based on previous inputs by the clerks or practitioners and rules within the various information systems.

4 Results

4A Results will be in a structured form. The use of SNOMED-CT to codify reports allows for the standardised sharing of information as well as aiding individual and group healthcare provision, owing to the simplicity of providing 'plain English' breakdowns (the codes can be expanded/translated as necessary).

4B Results will be interpreted manually. There are various automated routines that can be carried out on completed examinations to maximise throughput and minimise human effort at the result interpretation stage, with the most common being for standardised display protocols (DPs) to provide the optimal presentation for image interpretation in both radiology and pathology. The textual portion of the result can also be added quickly with the aid of standard templates, including pre-populated text or headings, plus with speech recognition available for digital dictation. This allows the reporting practitioner to see the result text and authorise immediately, minimising secretarial delays.

4C The initial results in the future may also be interpreted automatically. In addition to human generated reports, computer aided diagnosis (CAD) will be a more frequently used tool that can support those reporting studies. In radiology, currently this is possible for bone age assessments (CR/DDR), lung cancer (CT), breast cancer (mammography, MG), colon cancer (CT), prostate cancer (MR), and coronary heart disease (CT). In pathology, automatic cell counting and abnormality detection is a common CAD feature available. CAD is now developing other methods of machine learning, such as the automatic discovery of clinically relevant details, based on Multilayer Perceptron Artificial Neural Networks, Linear Discriminant Analysis and Quadratic Discriminant Analysis – fields of research that learn from a human's repeated choices and actions. This type of machine-based assistance could help highlight certain pathologies to both imaging and non-imaging staff before a formal 'human' report is produced, providing far more rapid feedback than is currently possible with retrospective peer review regimens.

4D Results will be available locally as a minimum requirement, within the healthcare organisation. The access to radiology information (ARI) IHE profile shares the study images throughout a single organisation, with the most common scenario allowing staff to access the PACS/image archive directly or via links within an EPR. MDT meetings could also use this approach along with a unified communications system, so that the whole team did not have to physically be in the same location.

4E Results will be available to other organisations that also care for the patient, enabling collaboration. Currently textual results may be sent as a HL7 message to systems that can receive them, with a 'read-receipt' returned as necessary. Implementing communications between PACS/ RIS, EPR/PHR and exchange systems will allow effective sharing of results in IHE profiles, such as the patient plan of care (PPOC). PPOC determines where data are exchanged relating to the creating and managing of individualised patient care – any results that are sent to a specific location should receive an acknowledgement that the results have been viewed, with a name, position, date/time, and possible contact details.

4F Results may be used for 3D printing for surgery or a variety of uses. Currently DICOM images can be converted to 3D printable medical models, and these can be used for education, patient counselling, training, and surgical planning (e.g. customised vessel stents used in angiography).

5 Result Distribution/Other Collaborative Steps

5A Patients will be able to track status updates and make amendments or update their own personal records if necessary. The patients via their PHR will be able to add notes to their record or provide other amendments for relevant healthcare staff to access, with alerting systems in place to identify worsening conditions recorded directly by the patient.

5B Data can be shared in a deidentified manner locally or internationally, as it will be coded via SNOMED-CT along with the results being in a structured form. This can be used for wider treatment of similar patient groups, plus for research (with a potential revenue for commercial licensing), by making this data available to both private and public organisations on an aggregated basis. These shared data, if used effectively, will transform healthcare systems by reducing costs and improving health outcomes by making healthcare planning more accurate – allowing for the targeting of personalised healthcare.

Above all, interoperability is just beginning to take shape in the UK, and it is noticeable that those in key departments, such as Radiology and Pathology, have a head start in shaping the direction for those in other departments.

CHAPTER 7

IMAGE REPORTING AND INTERPRETATION

Core Functions of Reporting

In addition to production of the actual report, many elements in the process of general reporting workflow need to be considered:

- Clinical decision support input.
- Display of the patient history and clinical problem.
- Initial informal commenting and alerting at the time of acquisition of the images.
- Reporting and productivity tools.
- Voice recognition and report input.
- Double and/or deadlock reporting.
- Formal alerting and clinical feedback.
- Self-education and teaching files (identified by keyword searching or in folders).

Informatics seeks to provide an efficient workflow with suitable tools to incorporate the above steps as seamlessly as possible. Anecdotally often this is not the case, with solutions to workflow problems focussing too heavily on specific tasks rather than the whole process from beginning to end.

The act of reporting imaging studies itself is usually carried out from pre-set worklists, configured in advance by the imaging informatics team. These worklists are dynamically updated according to a set of criteria (e.g. all unreported CT exams), which can either be hosted within the RIS, or now in modern systems, within the PACS. The use of worklists allows for fair distribution of reporting according to the reporter's clinical competencies, while maintaining a priority list if there is a significant backlog of reporting or if different areas have varying service level agreements/expectations.

Clinical Decision Support Input

It is unlikely that clinicians will be fully familiar with the vast array of guidelines and pathways for a given speciality (especially as developments in the field of medicine are continually ongoing), or even to find them rapidly during a short consultation session. CDS is customised software that guides a clinician through the best pathways for a given clinical problem. This aids the referring clinician in ensuring a patient is directed towards the most appropriate investigation(s) in a timely way, as well as ensuring that particular diagnostic specialities are not inappropriately overused. CDS makes decisions based on the combination of the relevant up-to-date guidelines, and integrates with other health systems to cross-correlate with, for example, blood results or medications. Utilising a CDS with interconnectivity into the imaging systems also allows reporting staff to see the initial preliminary steps already taken, leading to the clinical question required to be answered as part of the imaging examination in front of them, plus have options for potential differential diagnoses presented automatically. Owing to its relative newness, CDS is not yet widespread in the UK, but is found more extensively in the USA.

Patient History and Clinical Problem

Crucial for framing a high quality report, the patient history and clinical question to be answered must be conveyed from the referrer and be available without delay alongside the imaging for reference. Paperless solutions are obviously optimal for this (an OCS passing data to RIS, then displaying these fields in PACS alongside the relevant imaging is the current 'expected' solution). With this in mind, imaging itself has had good success with developing integration between its own systems; however, integration with other electronic health systems at the beginning (requesting/ordering) and the end (sending of reports/alerts/faxing) of the patient's journey through the Radiology department remains more challenging, with some paper processes persisting. Clinicians should also be encouraged to make use of any examination comments functionality in the PACS or OCS to feed back to reporting staff the disposal outcome of the patient episode (whether they felt there was a pathology/whether the patient was requested to return for follow-up). For example, in a trauma attendance if the reporter knows the patient has been referred to the fracture clinic rather than being simply sent home as 'normal', they will save time by not having to verify this if an otherwise subtle fracture is subsequently found on the images.

In the past, NHS England has repeatedly committed to complete EPRs, the latest date for this being imminent. What effect this will have in radiology is difficult to determine, as the remaining areas pertinent to the reporting process (the request made on paper and urgent report alerts sent by fax) are generally outside the control of the imaging informatics professionals who work within radiology. There are of course other internal paper-based systems that are difficult to easily convert to a paperless work flow: the consent form, the MRI safety questionnaire, the World Health Organization surgical checklist, the pregnancy status patient signature, each of which are currently scanned and stored as images. Despite best efforts to reduce paper usage, many departments currently struggle to move fully paperless in this area as the tendency to move back to paper is hard to resist, simply for its convenience at the point of acquisition (in practical terms, radiographers find it easier to work with light, flexible paper rather than heavier, inflexible tablet devices with a poor wifi connection in most situations).

Informal Commenting and Alerting at Acquisition

The value of alerting and commenting to the referrer at the time of acquisition is continually promoted in the UK, mainly as reporting backlogs and consequently time delay to a final report can vary dramatically. With targets, such as the 4-hour limit in A&E departments, being a well-publicised external measure of performance of a healthcare institution, there is an ever greater push on rapid progression through the patient journey. A shortage of appropriately trained staff and prioritising of certain types of studies sees the encouragement towards practitioners, such as radiographers, offering an informal comment as a means to reduce the time between imaging acquisition and findings being delivered. In practice, there are already a variety of methods for this – radiographers offering opinions via a template feedback sheet in A&E or radiology registrars writing a provisional report for multi-planar examinations out-of-hours. Advanced practitioners or specialist radiographers may also make notes in patient records during an ultrasound or barium exam or, at the very least, the ubiquitous 'red dot' (so called owing to the red circular stickers historically used on physical films for the purpose) or modern asterisk systems used in trauma scenarios, which indicate to inexperienced junior clinicians that there may be something amiss with an image by the placement of a trigger mark. These triggers may be supplemented by a note in either the PACS or RIS examination comments section to clarify the radiographer's observations.

However, poor mark placement on an image has the potential to influence inexperienced staff negatively – if a large arrow or a mark is placed next to an obvious pathology or fracture, human psychology (particularly in a rushed or busy environment) directs attention to this point and reduces the likelihood of other more subtle pathologies being observed in other areas of the image, or encourages the belief that an actual non-existent pathology does in fact exist. For this reason, it is recommended that trigger marks should only be placed at the corner of the image, not close to anatomy. An asterisk (*) in the top left or top right corner of the image (as appropriate given the anatomy and image placements) is recommended for this. It is also good practice to avoid the unnecessary use of text (e.g. 'red dot') in order to reduce confusion if the images are viewed subsequently outside of the UK (either as part of the patient's journey or for out-sourced backlog reporting) and also to prevent patient concern if they view the image incidentally. A '#' fracture symbol is also not recommended for this purpose as it references numerals rather than pathologies outside of the UK.

Reporting and Productivity Tools

A commonly used reporting setup is shown in **Fig. 7.1**. The basic user will be familiar with the standard everyday functions in image viewing

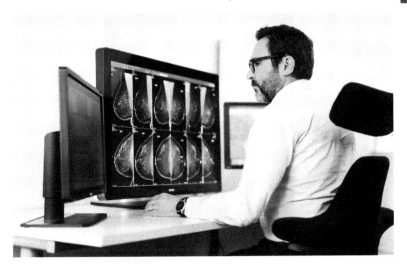

Fig. 7.1 Typical reporting station setup.

applications, such as window, zoom, edge enhancement, invert, crop, measure, and angle. Perhaps less familiar are functions such as cardiothoracic ratio measurement tools, spine labelling, NM volume of interest, density unit indicators, and measurement of areas of varying shapes. Each modality also has its own unique set of add-on tools, which are custom designed to the outputs of that imaging speciality. In the same way, each member of reporting staff has their own favourite and combination of tools, which they prefer to use. Some systems also incorporate the addition of mixed ologies – with medical photography images, cardiology studies, ECGs, and other information presented alongside imaging in order to provide a simple single source for diagnostic material. Presenting medical information in this manner is nontraditional but provides a rich bed of source material for those offering opinions as part of their reports. Key image functionality is also useful for the clinician's later use following reporting – radiology images can consist of thousands of slices, and referencing those that are referred to in a report provides a time-saving reference for referrers.

Computer Aided Diagnosis/Computer Aided Detection. CAD provides automated analysis of an image or series utilising either pre-set or

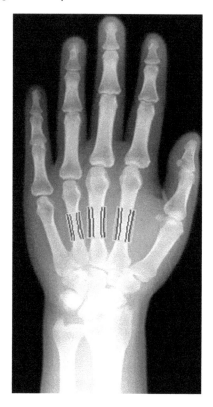

Fig. 7.2 Automated osteoporosis detection overlaid onto clinical imaging.

machine-led learning algorithms to generate a diagnostic opinion independently of the human operator. This is commonly used for bone age or osteoporosis assessments, lung, breast, colon and prostate cancer, coronary heart disease, and for automatic cell counting in pathological specimens. CAD results are typically toggled on and off by the human reporter after they have made an initial assessment of the image, but before they finalise their opinion. The input that CAD provides into reports maximises the accuracy of pathological detection. **Figure 7.2** shows automated osteoporosis detection overlays on clinical images.

Voice Recognition

Voice (speech) recognition (VR) is considered an obligatory part of expedient radiology reporting in the UK, with every major acute site in England utilising some form of this technology to decrease report turnaround times while increasing throughput.

There are two main voice recognition programs in use across the UK at present, both manufactured by the same vendor and carrying the brand names SpeechMagic/SpeechAnywhere and Dragon. Although they are separate applications currently, the technology underpinning their functionality is being merged by the vendor, so there is little other differentiation available in this area aside from user interfaces and programmability differences. The best quality recognition is obtained from extensive initial training (a series of texts are read to the machine in order that it can adapt to the user's individual voice by comparing the sound and tone to the words and pronunciation actually expected and anticipated by the software) in addition to acoustic adaption (a short passage read to the machine by each user prior to reporting at a new workstation in order to calibrate to any background noises that differ across reporting locations). These two learning processes are extremely important for high recognition rates; however, as they are fairly time consuming and less interesting to complete, many users attempt to skip or work through them in an unnaturally fast manner resulting in permanently inferior recognition. As a result of the need for voice profiles, individual accounts are required – accounts cannot be shared – making licensing potentially expensive, and a reason why some reporting staff, such as sonographers, are occasionally excluded from licensing arrangements and use of VR. Many sites experience ongoing problems with VR, particularly with corrupt voice profiles (the files that store a user's pronunciation templates for the software to use) meaning regular backups and reinforcement of good working practices is required (logging off and switching users cleanly). Anecdotally, as VR software has been in existence for several decades it is comparatively well developed – even deaf individuals or those with strong accents can find a manner in which the software will operate for them.

However, in some cases, there is still a need for third party specialist transcription rather than VR. This may be in surgical cases (where a microphone cannot be held or worn, but a ceiling microphone can pick up enough detail for humans to listen and discern the person dictating rather than the other individuals around them), or where certain physiological conditions produce a greatly non-standard speaking pattern for some individuals.

Desktop integration. Historically, the systems displaying images and text have been separate. DTI reduces the risk associated with having two different clinical systems open (the risk of inadvertently selecting different patients in each) and also introduces the convenience of synchronisation, whereby if a reporting list is navigated within PACS, the associated RIS entries automatically keep pace in another application, saving time and operator intervention. DTI can also be combined with single sign-on functionality, where one login is sufficient to authenticate access into multiple systems.

Report Input: Templates (Stock Text)

Reports can either be entered beginning with a blank screen, or by the insertion of several appropriate preformatted paragraphs, which reporters add to or adapt. In many cases, such as complex MR or NM bone densitometry examinations, it is judicious to have these common sentences ('stock text') or indeed whole paragraphs prepared – primarily for the ease of interpretation and review by clinicians as the data are presented in a standard reproducible format, but also for time saving purposes and to prevent any conclusions being missed from the report.

As reporting staff progress through their career they begin to amass a library of stock texts and paragraphs. These may be stored in something as simple as a text file where portions are cut from and pasted into an imaging report as appropriate, or inserted by a pre-determined keyboard shortcut key combination or even by voice macros (dictating a specific trigger phrase, perhaps 'command report normal chest', to trigger insertion of a much longer sentence/paragraph). Some reports can be pre-populated from system measurements, e.g. percentage stenosis values of blood vessels or bone density measurements.

Structured Reporting

Some organisations prefer to utilise fixed reporting templates that require the reporter to answer specific questions in order, e.g. making comparisons with prior studies, commenting on technique or quality of the imaging, providing an affirmative conclusion and suggestions for further suitable diagnostic studies or treatment. This is similar to filling out a form.

Double and Deadlock Reporting

Double reporting is particularly useful for some sensitive high accuracy workflows or for reporting staff competency checks. This is simply where a second author 'blindly' (i.e. without sight of the first report) reports the study with a second report, then they or another individual compares that second opinion to the first author's report. In case of a disagreement, a third reporter is called to produce a 'deadlock' report. The deadlock reporter may or may not have sight of the conflicting reports prior to forming their opinion.

Double reading, discordance, and arbitration. A specialist type of image 'reading' used in MG reporting, two staff members scrutinise the images and either agree or disagree a categorisation. If there is no agreement (a 'discordant result'), a third member of reporting staff acts as arbitrator.

Alerting and Clinical Feedback

At present, manual fax, telephone, or email notifications are the most common method of alerting the referrer for urgent findings (cancers, initially unnoticed fracture requiring patient recall, etc.). Systems that allow the automated notifications and requiring acknowledgments with reminders if no action is taken within a certain time period are available, but not widely used. Organisations, such as the Royal College of Radiologists, have indicated this as a persistent risk with imaging informatics equipment.

In addition to the issues with alerting, as mentioned by our clinical colleagues in a later chapter, there is presently no single widespread method for feedback on imaging reports (quality, accuracy, or usefulness) to reach the original reporter in the UK. Likewise, there are only complicated pathways for those radiographers acquiring the imaging or reporting staff providing the reports to follow-up on the patient's actual condition or further findings.

There are also practical issues, particularly with informal commenting; if the study has an initial report authored by a trainee (which by its nature will be reviewed by a senior), the senior has authored a change, there has then been sub-speciality input for a third change, plus potentially a fourth version of the report exists following a MDT meeting. By convention, all report versions after the initial are addended (added one after another) rather than the original changed or removed, and therefore a study could possibly have three or more reports assigned to it, presenting an opportunity for misinterpretation at the destination, particularly if time passes between report versions. Red dot indications added by radiographers may not prove immediately useful if there are no accompanying notes to identify the concern, or if they are placed inappropriately.

Self-Education and Teaching Files

Experience and continuing professional development is key for those carrying out reporting duties. As an increasing number of institutions now have greater than 50% of extremity 'plain films' reported by AHP, plus other areas (such as barium swallow investigations reported by speech and language therapists, and trauma studies by nurse practitioners), it is now critical that learning opportunities are available across the enterprise, rather than constrained to a single group of staff.

Modern Imaging Informatics Processes

Teaching file tags. Unlike the 'old days' where boxes of slides were found hoarded under radiologists' desks for reference during 1:2:1 teaching sessions, modern PACS allows for cross-enterprise sharing by the 'tagging' of images, allowing for a simple search under the required keyword (pathology, body part, or condition) to locate cases others may have added as resources.

MDTs. These typically require different image presentation layouts to those required for standard clinical use of images; a method for keeping these separate from each other encourages planning and preparation. The ability to save notes from the sessions separately from clinical care notes is also a benefit.

Collaboration tools. Unified communications (e.g. Skype) video call integration, email, SMS capabilities, and live chat with image sharing save time on visiting other offices or relaying patient identifiers via telephone when consultations with other colleagues are required.

Personal worklists. Either for speciality reporting or for teaching purposes, these are separate from clinical workflows and can be customised as the individual's learning needs change (perhaps as the reporting staff member reports ever more complex material throughout their career).

Educational sharing. Connectivity with neighbouring institutions, particularly those with different or greater sub-speciality experience, is important and fairly straightforward with modern systems. There are now multiple ways of importing and exporting images while anonymising or retaining the patient demographics. Now a common PACS feature, auto-anonymised image exports straight into presentation software aids with the education of neighbouring sites and completion of discrepancy meetings. Internationally maintained teaching case websites exist and are widely used.

Performance monitoring. Dashboard systems showing concordance of opinion between reporting staff are helpful in identifying areas of weakness (or for refresher training) in reporting staff who would otherwise be working unsupervised.

Peer review. Closely linked to the above, peer review is the concept of 'voluntary' double reporting, allowing for feedback from peers or those with greater experience in reporting certain studies. Peer review is a form of quality assurance (QA) on the human output of radiology reporting.

CHAPTER 8
DICOM

DICOM is the internationally accepted standard used for storing, exchanging, and transmitting medical image data: by agreeing and unifying on a common standard a 'mixed-vendor' environment is possible. Its features include image storage, retrieval, and display (today on monitors, in previous years via printing).

History and Development

In the early 1980s, as each manufacturer utilised proprietary encoding for images it became apparent that it was difficult for medical imaging to be viewed or stored outside of the boundaries of the original acquisition modality, and indeed as a result of this some hospitals were forced into purchasing all equipment from a single manufacturer. Recognising a need for greater co-ordination between the different vendors and systems in the developing area of imaging informatics, groups began to debate the possible solutions. In 1985, the initial DICOM specification was first published jointly by the National Electrical Manufacturers Association (NEMA) and the American College of Radiology (ACR), with the aim of allowing interoperability. Today, several decades later, the third version of DICOM remains in use and is now backed up by a standard of the International Standard Organisation (ISO 12052:2006).

Viewing the most recent DICOM standard is free and easily accessible on the internet via the NEMA website. The current version of DICOM in use from 1993 onwards remains DICOM v3, which is still being developed, receiving regular updates but retaining the same version number. This is because all current updates are forwards and backwards compatible within the version, allowing for wide ranging compatibility between old and new equipment, even when recent technologies had not been foreseen originally, such as Bluetooth connected DDR imaging plates. A consequence of this interoperability is that an estimated trillion (a thousand billion) medical images can be viewed and transferred with DICOM today, unlike other formats, which have peaked and waned over the same timeframe (would you be able to open a previously common Microsoft Works or Word Perfect document from a floppy disk in your hospital now?). Older equipment, such as legacy NM scanners, can also happily co-exist on a network with cutting-edge volume reconstruction or image analysis packages. To reduce confusion, the DICOM standard is defined as the sum of all approved parts, supplements, and agreed change proposals – there are no distinct revisions (v.3.17 etc.) and changes are rolled into a new edition periodically. In the field, PACS professionals tend to refer to DICOM revisions by year of revision, such as DICOM v3 2017, although this is not encouraged by NEMA.

The Function of DICOM

DICOM itself (as a standard) contains a number of parts, with 18 (20 total, with two retired) as of 2017. DICOM documents and defines a standard way for data to be formatted, communicated, and presented by medical imaging systems during the creation, management, and exchange of those images. By creating a common standard this allows imaging acquired on one manufacturer's device to be viewed on another compatible device much more widely, and is the basis for how we are able to 'mix-and-match' different pieces of equipment within our departments.

The standard overall defines:

- A set of protocols (rules) for manufacturers to use.
- The syntax (arrangement) and semantics (meaning) of commands and data models (relationships).
- Guidance on standardised formatting of data.
- Communication methods.

The various parts of the standard deal with each portion of the image handling process. Key functionality is explained below, and for comprehensive up-to-date technical details the requisite NEMA documents should be consulted online. As it is intentionally fairly wide reaching, the DICOM standard covers all medical imaging equipment (including PACS, RIS, MPI, workstations, and image acquisition stations). An interesting consequence of the need to be backward compatible is that portions of the DICOM standard still include the requirement for modalities to be compatible with what we would today consider to be antiquated technologies, such as the predecessors of standard networks (which were still available in the 1990s), or even film printers.

Common DICOM Terms

Terms commonly used for DICOM are shown in *Table 8.1*.

Modality

In correct terminology, a modality is a discrete type of imaging speciality, such as CT, MR, CR, and US; however, in popular usage it is used (incorrectly) to refer to a single acquisition station.

AETs

A common term in the PACS Office, AETs are the 'names' of services or applications communicating within the network, typically used to identify individual pieces of image acquisition equipment. Similar to a mailbox address, these must be locally unique within the same network,

Table 8.1 Common DICOM terms and simplifications

DICOM term	Simplification
Application entity	Person
Association	Conversation
SOP class	Topic of conversation
SOP instance	Piece of information
Transfer syntax	Language
Service	Form of conversation (lecture, question and answer, reference sheet, etc.)
Off-line media	Printed book
AET	Person's name

AET, application entity title; DICOM, digital imaging and communications in medicine; SOP, service-object pair.

with a maximum length of 16 characters. It is good practice within the UK to ensure AETs used in each hospital are prefixed with the site ODS code. This aids image sharing (as PACS worklists can then be quickly built to include an AET or station name or exclude 'foreign' AETs as desired) and for future-proofing, as hospitals become increasingly joined up.

Modality Worklists

A DICOM service that provides a collated feed of demographic and exam data to image acquisition equipment. This is typically filtered by a selective query to display only relevant exams for a certain examination room and then sorted by attendance date/time for ease of reference and selection by the operators of that equipment.

Query/Retrieve

The query/retrieve (Q/R) service provides a method to search (query) for particular attributes – normally a patient name, patient ID, or date of birth, etc., then to download (retrieve) the matching examination data and images. Workstations make great use of this when bringing images for display on reporting terminals. The national Image Exchange Portal utilises Q/R to search for matching patients when demographics are entered on the transfer or request sections of the system.

Association

A connection or conversation between two programs is known as an association. Associations are generally short lived rather than being maintained constantly for extended periods, owing to each program having a maximum number of associations that can take place at any one time. The DICOM standard uses the transmission control protocol/internet protocol (TCP/IP) communications protocol to communicate between systems over a network, with port 104 being assigned most commonly.

SOP Class

Service-object pair (SOP) class is effectively equivalent to the 'topic' of a conversation and is framed in context with the actor ('thing' doing the action) plus the action required.

SCU/SCP

Service class user (SCU) and service class provider (SCP) are simply the two 'ends' of a single connection at any one time – the SCU is the end initiating the contact, and the SCP the receiver or responder, just in the same manner as humans initiate two-way conversations in pairs – one person asks a question, the other listens, then answers.

Composite and Normalised Operations

Composite operations (beginning with C-) are found as part of wider sets of instructions, whereas normalised operations (beginning with N-) contain enough information to be free-standing as a single instruction. In standard use, composite operations account for many of the DICOM file operations observed on the front-end of the PACS as they are issued in context with other surrounding instructions to form a required set of actions (it is rare for an acquisition station to simply say, 'here, have this image', without context).

Basic DICOM File Movement Operations

- *C-Store:* send data for storage. As a safety check, a service known as storage commitment (SCM) can check that there is sufficient space prior to the operation beginning, and at the end that the data have actually been stored before the sending program discards the data (this avoids an equivalent of the common issue found on standard operating systems where a file copies for several minutes, before an 'out of memory' message is displayed).

- C-*Find:* search for something and return results.
- C-*Move:* copy a composite object in a new, following, association (that composite object is usually a DICOM image, but can be other rarer items).
- C-*Get:* also copies a composite object, but without starting a new association to do so.
- C-*Echo:* similar to a 'ping', this checks the low-level technical operation of the connection and destination application.

Other operations, including normalised operations, do exist and are listed in the respective DICOM standard part.

The simplified basic process for establishing connections in DICOM is for the *SCU* (entity wanting something done) to communicate with the *SCP* (entity that can likely do this), firstly *negotiating* a technical protocol (mutually as fast as possible, but understandable language) leading to an *association* (a conversation) being created. Through this association, the requests are made and data are passed (using the *composite operations* above, or perhaps the normalised operations, as so needed). The association is then closed.

Conformance Statements

DICOM conformance statements are important but extremely lengthy documents issued for each piece of equipment, such as a PACS, CR console, CT scanner, which detail in depth the particular machine's specific compliance and implementation of the DICOM standard. This is needed, as although the overall DICOM version has remained unchanged for years at version 3, additional functionality and methods have been added. Reading the conformance statement of any new incoming piece of imaging equipment is critically important to determine any compatibility or workflow issues that may arise. This review should be carried out well in advance of a purchasing decision being made by those in charge of managing the PACS in conjunction with the department lead wishing to purchase or add new equipment.

Modality Performed Procedure Step

A useful DICOM service, but not widely adopted within the radiology community at present, modality performed procedure step (MPPS) allows for feedback to be sent from the image acquisition station such that individual parts of the diagnostic examinations can be sent separately, and the status of these updated, also separately. For example, a 'progress' update can be made on multi-body-part examinations with earlier images then being made available for review more quickly than the entire examination; or staged dose information provided. This partially provides similar functionality to the historic requests for 'wet film' images (clinicians requiring to see chemically-developed radiographs as soon as they were removed from the development process).

Composite Instances

Meaning 'a part of more than one', by far the most common composite instance is the DICOM image (examined in more detail shortly). Some others are:

- Presentation states: contain a record of adjustments or manipulations made to a diagnostic image, such that the original image is not affected, and the presentation state (changes) can be toggled at will in entirety.
- Radiotherapy objects: similar to DICOM images produced as the output to diagnostic encounters, but without pixel data (images), instead containing radiotherapy dose and planning information, etc.
- Structured reports: a 'framework' for issuing reports in a reproducible manner (similar to each report being from a template).

The DICOM File

Formally known as 'DICOM data objects', these consist of a number of attributes (components), including a preamble (identifying the file type and components), a block of data (commonly known as the DICOM headers, comprising patient demographics, technical information about the image, the study, its acquisition parameters, and acquisition device together with many other listed attributes), and the image data itself (a single attribute that holds the data required to recreate the image pixels or voxels).

The DICOM Header

Each image generated by medical equipment has, stored within it, a chunk of information about the technical aspects of the image, the patient, and the transfer methods at its start, followed by the actual image data. An example, using a fictitious patient, is illustrated in **Fig. 8.1**.

This screen can look quite complex and daunting at first, but dissecting each line is possible just by reading across one row at a time. A sample DICOM tag would read:

0008 0020 | 8 | study_date | DA | 1 | "20130415"

In this example, the two blocks of hexadecimal characters (all numerical here) at the start of each row are the *Group* and *Element* number – these reference parts of the standard and help equipment know what information is being presented. *Length* advises the maximum size of the value. Next, the *Description* aids human interpretation by providing the short explanation of the row. Following this are the *Value Representation (VR)* and *Value Multiplicity (VM)* figures; the VR provides the type of value the system should expect to find (e.g. DT = Date and Time; UI = Unique Identifier; TM = time) from a list contained within the DICOM standard. The VM then indicates how many values are provided. Finally the actual **value** is given. Lists of all public groups, elements, and possible VR/VM options are given in the DICOM data structures and encoding document. Note that dates as utilised in DICOM are stored in the international format: YYYYMMDD to avoid the need to convert between respective USA and UK formats.

UIDs

Several unique identifiers (UIDs) are generated within each modality and are included within the produced images. These identifiers together serve to present different information about the generating devices, the patient, the individual encounter, and the files making up the study. Continuing this, each image within a study contains a number of different UIDs in order to link that single image to the remainder of the series, the exam, and the overall patient encounter (the hierarchy being: Patient > Study > Series > Image). UIDs generated as part of the process are intended to be globally unique and

Grp	Elmt	Length	Description	VR	VM	Value
0008	0005	10	specific_character_set	CS	1-n	"ISO_IR 100"
0008	0008	34	image_type	CS	1-n	"ORIGINAL\PRIMARY\AXIAL\CT_SOM5 SEQ"
0008	0016	26	sop_class_uid	UI	1	"1.2.840.10008.5.1.4.1.1.2"
0008	0018	56	sop_instance_uid	UI	1	"1.3.12.2.1107.5.1.4.54168.30000013041507523079600001239"
0008	0020	8	study_date	DA	1	"20130415"
0008	0021	8	series_date	DA	1	"20130415"
0008	0022	8	acquisition_date	DA	1	"20130415"
0008	0023	8	image_date	DA	1	"20130415"
0008	0030	14	study_time	TM	1	"113931.812000"
0008	0031	14	series_time	TM	1	"113931.812000"
0008	0032	14	acquisition_time	TM	1	"114006.015408"
0008	0033	14	image_time	TM	1	"114006.015408"
0008	0050	12	accession_number	SH	1	"100000794862"
0008	0060	2	modality	CS	1	"CT"
0008	0070	8	manufacturer	LO	1	"SIEMENS"
0008	0080	24	institution_name	LO	1	"ROYAL BROMPTON HOSPITAL"

Fig. 8.1 Overview of a DICOM header.

A Section of DICOM header (each row gives one DICOM tag)

UIDs

Grp	Elmt	Length	Description	VR	VM	Value
0008	0005	10	specific_character_set	CS	1-n	"ISO_IR 100"
0008	0008	34	image_type	CS	1-n	"ORIGINAL\PRIMARY\AXIAL\CT_SOM5 SEQ"
0008	0016	26	sop_class_uid	UI	1	"1.2.840.10008.5.1.4.1.1.2"
0008	0018	56	sop_instance_uid	UI	1	"1.3.12.2.1107.5.1.4.54168.30000013041507523079600001239"
0008	0020	8	study_date	DA	1	"20130415"
0008	0021	8	series_date	DA	1	"20130415"
0008	0022	8	acquisition_date	DA	1	"20130415"
0008	0023	8	image_date	DA	1	"20130415"
0008	0030	14	study_time	TM	1	"113931.812000"
0008	0031	14	series_time	TM	1	"113931.812000"
0008	0032	14	acquisition_time	TM	1	"114006.015408"
0008	0033	14	image_time	TM	1	"114006.015408"
0008	0050	12	accession_number	SH	1	"100000794862"
0008	0060	2	modality	CS	1	"CT"
0008	0070	8	manufacturer	LO	1	"SIEMENS"
0008	0080	24	institution_name	LO	1	"ROYAL BROMPTON HOSPITAL"

Fig. 8.2 UIDs within a DICOM header. (VM, value multiplicity; VR, value representation.)

there are various issuing registries, which seek to avoid duplication by assigning batches to manufacturers and individuals or sites as required. UIDs generated for DICOM services all begin with the leading digits 1.2.840.10008[…] allowing for their easy recognition among wider network traffic. **Figure 8.2** identifies UIDs within a portion of a sample DICOM header.

Public Tags versus Private Tags

Public Tags

As shown in **Fig. 8.3**, public tags are the 'common' tags that have been internationally standardised by committee and are likely to be found in normal circumstances. These range from being common in every exam (patient name, date of birth, address, accession number, etc.), to those only found in certain examinations (e.g. pitch, scan width, slice thickness in CT). Public tags have even group numbers (the first block of numbers on each row, such as [0008], [0010]).

Private Tags

Private tags found in medical image headers are differentiated from public tags by their group numbers being odd numbers (**Fig. 8.4**).

Private tags contain pieces of image information that are either unique to the equipment through which the image was acquired, or are extra pieces of data provided beyond that available in public tags to allow for more speciality use. Some uses of private tags may create a form of vendor lock-in – a problem historically seen within

```
0008 1030     12 | study_description                  |LO| 1 | "12 Lead ECG"
0008 103e     20 | series_description                 |LO| 1 | "HRCT_Expiration 1/10"
0008 1040      8 | institutional_department_name      |LO| 1 | "DEFAULT"
0008 1090     12 | manufacturer_model_name            |LO| 1 | "Sensation 64"
0010 0010     26 | patient_name                       |PN| 1 | "SMITH^JONATHAN^^"
0010 0020      6 | patient_id                         |LO| 1 | "123456"
0010 0030      8 | patient_birth_date                 |DA| 1 | "19010101"
0010 0040      2 | patient_sex                        |CS| 1 | "M"
0010 1010      4 | patient_age                        |AS| 1 | "120Y"
0010 1030      4 | patient_weight                     |DS| 1 | "52.8"
```

Fig. 8.3 A selection of the more common public tags.

```
0011 1036         4 | Unknown element | DS | ? | "656"
0011 1037        18 | Unknown element | DS | ? | "-5.0\-3.0\2.0\4.0"
0011 1042        16 | Unknown element | LO | ? | "antero-posterior"
0011 1044        16 | Unknown element | CS | ? | "DIGITALCASSETTE"
0011 1046        52 | Unknown element | LO | ? | "Chest\antero-posterior\Standard\MEDIUM ADULT\Custom1"
0011 1047        10 | Unknown element | DS | ? | "798.940247"
0011 1059         6 | Unknown element | CS | ? | "NORMAL"
0011 1064        12 | Unknown element | CS | ? | "URP_DETECTOR"
0011 1066         2 | Unknown element | CS | ? | "No"
0011 1067         4 | Unknown element | CS | ? | "None"
0011 1068        16 | Unknown element | CS | ? | "40:f4:a0:0:bc:b4"
0011 1069        10 | Unknown element | CS | ? | "-1.000000"
0011 106b     32768 | Unknown element | US | ? | 0x0000 0 ...
0011 106d        18 | Unknown element | DS | ? | "217.308115523737311"
0011 1076         4 | Unknown element | CS | ? | "L\F"
0011 107d         2 | Unknown element | CS | ? | "NO"
0011 107e         2 | Unknown element | DS | ? | "0"
0011 1080         2 | Unknown element | DS | ? | "2"
0011 1081         2 | Unknown element | LO | ? | "AP"
0011 1082        18 | Unknown element | CS | ? | "GRID_FREQ_70_LP_CM"
```

Fig. 8.4 A selection of private tags.

CT – without knowledge of the specific private tags and expected data held within them it may only be possible to efficiently use a reconstruction station of the same brand (and perhaps even model line) as the acquiring CT scanner.

Photometric Interpretations

Not all digital images are captured solely in greyscale; even when images are in greyscale there is a question as to which 'way-around' the greyscale is applied in a particular image. For example, in a greyscale range of 0–256, is 0 the whitest pixel value with 256 being pure black (a gradient of grey shades between) or vice versa? Defining the photometric interpretation is carried out with every image and allows display software to render (display) images faithfully as intended. During 2013, problems with incorrect photometric interpretation values were found, with legacy CR equipment images being displayed inverted when transmitted through data sharing services until a patch for the original equipment was applied. Photometric interpretation values are typically: Monochrome 2 (the lowest pixel value is displayed black), Monochrome 1 (the lowest pixel value is displayed white) or RGB (colour for display on monitors). A photometric interpretation DICOM tag is included in every image to ensure images display correctly.

Viewing DICOM Images Outside of PACS

To view individual DICOM images away from the medical environment where the original PACS viewer is not available, a dedicated program can be used to open the files (e.g. either Osirix for the Mac environment, or DICOMworks for Microsoft Windows-based PCs). Some operating systems also include native support (Windows 7, but not 10), meaning that opening DICOM imaging is as simple as opening a standard JPEG photo in these. It must be remembered that DICOM files do contain the patient demographics and episode details embedded within their header information – thorough de-identification of teaching cases is very important to preserve confidentiality, particularly when working with images containing a large number of private tags that may contain 'hidden' duplicate demographics not removed by the automated anonymisation techniques.

In daily practice, images viewed away from a PACS environment are typically presented on what is known as 'offline media'. This term in this context refers to the CDs and DVDs we have become so familiar with, containing the DICOM files, a viewing application, and possibly other files. Offline media, such as CDs/DVDs, exported from PACS need to have a structure table formed according to the DICOM standard, commonly in the form of a DICOMDIR file in the root directory (first folder of the media). The DICOMDIR file is simply an index of the images, containing the hierarchical structure of the examination (Patient > Study > Series > Image) and setting out the relation between each of the images on that disk in order for them to be displayed correctly. Without this file, some current PACS may not be able to import the studies as the hierarchy may not be automatically recoverable without manual intervention.

Cross-Enterprise Document Sharing for Imaging

Within radiology, the standards widely used for storing and transferring textual and image data are HL7 and DICOM, respectively. However, there are so many different vendors and implementations of radiology PACS and RIS (not to mention EPR, MPI, OCS, etc.) that the IHE initiative was launched by vendors and healthcare professionals to improve the sharing of healthcare data between systems that have the same function (but perhaps different vendors, layouts, or stylistic differences). IHE created an interoperability profile (detailed specification) named XDS or, specifically for Radiology departments, XDS-I. These profiles simply recommend methods for the technical manners of sharing via interconnections between different healthcare systems and organisations, many of which use different vendors, albeit for the same task. XDS allows for the creation of a centralised list of studies across a wide area (and multiple radiology systems) meaning it is being found as a solution to the problem facing many institutions of not knowing where a

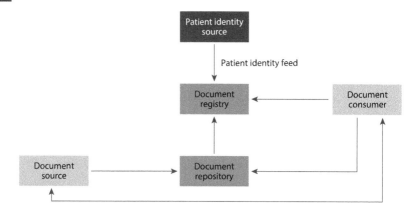

Fig. 8.5 XDS overview.

patient was last imaged externally (outside their own boundaries). However, as of 2017, XDS is not yet widely used in radiology owing to it being relatively newly launched, but it is gaining popularity as the next generation of PACS and Enterprise Archives are being installed in the late 2010s. XDS complements HL7 and DICOM standards by providing the facility to centrally register documents against a patient, and distribute and provide access to them without necessarily making copies.

XDS itself is designed for multiple applications within healthcare, and so a 'document' refers to a diagnostic image (an X-ray or CT scan etc.) in this context. The interoperability profile is designed to reduce the need for duplicating or copying images across the country, reducing the risk to patients that subsequently outdated copies of imaging are incorrectly relied upon during treatment.

An overview of XDS is shown in **Fig. 8.5**.

Principles of XDS-I

Patient Registry

XDS allows users (the document 'consumers') to search for all relevant documents for a specific patient by building up an index (register) of the documents as they are acquired for each patient.

Patient Identity Source

Before a document can be registered against a patient the system needs to know about the patient. The usual source for patient demographics in NHS hospitals, either directly or indirectly, is the MPI, potentially via a PAS or RIS.

Document Repository

Simply stores the documents (or the 'KOS object' for DICOM images) that are registered. More than one document repository can exist.

KOS Object

KOS objects are items with an index of pointers to DICOM studies, series, and instances for a patient. They point to where images are held and contain data on size, format, etc.

Document Source

Can be any compliant system that generates documents or images, like acquisition modalities.

Document Consumer

Any compliant system that can query the registry, retrieve from the repository, and display the document or images, such as an open-source or vendor neutral or traditional proprietary viewer. A typical XDS-I configuration is illustrated in **Fig. 8.6**.

A central XDS registry and repository is hosted within a location-agnostic datacentre. Patients are listed in the registry using data from the MPI of each healthcare institution. When a patient attendance in an imaging department is made on the RIS it is also registered in the central registry and its data stored in the central repository. Following the patient's imaging, the KOS object (pointers to images from the study in this case) is stored and indexed followed by the report document later. Using a web-based login, users then are able to have rapid access to radiology data across numerous Trusts, removing the problem of needing to create uncontrolled copies and duplicate data between sites.

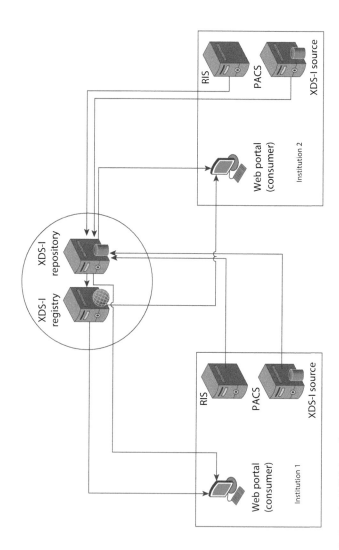

Fig. 8.6 A typical XDS-I configuration. (PACS, picture archiving and communication system; RIS, radiology information system; XDS-I, cross-enterprise document sharing for imaging.)

HL7

Unlike DICOM, HL7 is a closed commercialised standard maintained by the Health Level Seven International Organisation, and until late 2013 was completely unavailable for quick review on the internet without paid membership of the organisation. Today, the standards are available for download, but only for personal use – the standard remains guarded, again in contrast to DICOM.

History and Development

HL7 itself was a standard born out of the need for connectivity and integration to enable the exchange of textual healthcare information to the benefit of patients. Originally developed from a predecessor research standard in the 1970s, it was first used more widely in university or development settings from 1981 onwards. HL7 v2 was published in late 1989 and is continually updated, with the minor version numbers changing.

Different versions of HL7 are available for use today:

- HL7 version 3 is less commonly used, and is infrequently encountered in the 'normal' imaging environment – it utilises a more user-friendly XML layout, meaning it has increased uptake in the newer fields of use, such as medication management, prescription ordering, dietetics, some laboratory systems, and GP electronic records, but because of the long-standing historic use of the dissimilar version 2 in other areas has not seen universal adoption;

- HL7 version 2 is the most commonly used version of the standard. Newer releases within version 2 are backwards compatible and simply add on additional functionality, e.g. to enable integration to newly developed services, or incorporate new modernised workflows. Version 2.8.2 is the latest version available at the time of press.

HL7 is named after its position in the 7-layer OSI model by the ISO (**Fig. 9.1** and *Table 9.1*).

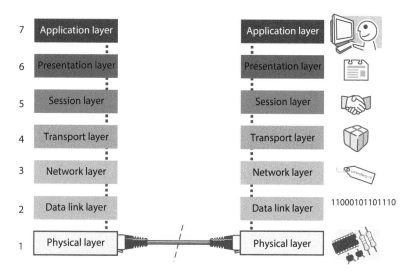

Fig. 9.1 The 7-layer OSI model.

Table 9.1 Examples of the 7 layers

Layer	Controls	Example
7	Application	HTTP, Telnet, DHCP, HL7
6	Presentation	MIME, XDR
5	Session	NetBIOS
4	Transport	TCP, UDP
3	Network	IP (v.4, v.6)
2	Data link	IEEE 802.3
1	Physical	USB, Bluetooth, Wifi A, B, G, N, AB; Cat5e, Cat6 cabling

The remainder of this chapter discusses HL7 version 2, as the majority of imaging systems within the UK utilise this and will continue to do so for the foreseeable future.

The Function of HL7

HL7 messages are text strings, formatted in very specific, defined, repeatable ways.

Each message has every possible 'field' either filled or left empty, separated by specific characters (known as delimiters). All possible data types for particular fields are defined by the standard. Version 2 HL7 messages are intended for machine use and interpretation, rather than human manipulation.

Inside a HL7 Message

HL7 messages comprise separate segments, each prefixed with a standard code to indicate what type of information they hold. Reading the initial three characters of each new line in the sample message of **Fig. 9.2**, each segment is explained.

MSH

This segment contains *message header* information such as:

■ Message delimiters (characters such as |^~\&, which therefore cannot be used elsewhere in the HL7 message text – particularly important to remember for the ampersand – for instance, 'A&E' is not permitted without modification in a HL7 message).

```
MSH|^~\&|MegaReg|DSNHSFT|ImgOrdMgr|RadImgCtr|20170115090131-
    0500||ADT^A01|01052901|P|2.8.2
EVN|201701150901||||20170150900
PID|||56782445^^^UAReg^PI~999855750^^^USSSA^SS||ATKINSONTEST^JAMES
    ^A^JNR||19800910|M||2028-9^^HL70005^RA9999^^XYZ|12ASEASHORE ROAD
    ^^NEWPORT^DEVON^SS10 3AA^^H|||||||0105I30001^^^99DEF^AN
PV1|||W^389^1^UABH^^^^3||||1234567890^THILAKENDRAN^SUJENTHAR^S^^^MD^0010^UAMC^L||
    0123456789^MORTON^LINDSEY^A^^^MD^0010^UAMC^L|MED|||||A0|||13579^
    HODGKINSON^JENNA^A^^^MD^0010^UAMC^L
OBX|1|NM|^Body Height||1.85|m^Meter^ISO+|||||F
OBX|2|NM|^Body Weight||85|kg^Kilogram^ISO+|||||F
AL1|1||^CONTRAST AGENT
```

Fig. 9.2 A sample version 2 HL7 message. (HL7, health level 7.)

- Origin and destination.
- Date and time.
- Message type (here, ADT) and trigger event (here, A01).
- Message control ID.
- Processing ID.
- Version ID.

EVN

The EVN segment contains *event* information, such as:

- When the event was recorded.
- When the event occurred.
- Who was responsible.
- The event name.

PID

The PID segment contains current *patient identification* information:

- Identifiers.
- Names and addresses.
- Date/time of birth.
- Gender, ethnic origin.
- Account numbers.

PV1

This segment contains *patient visit* information, such as:

- Class (I/P or O/P).
- Doctors (attending, consulting, referring, admitting).
- Admit and discharge date and time.

OBX

An OBX segment contains *observation* information including:

- Data type of the observation.
- Name of the attribute being observed.
- Value and units.
- Observation status (such as preliminary or final).

AL1

The AL1 segment contains *allergy* information, such as:

- Severity.
- Type.

Just as with DICOM, dates in HL7 messages are formatted in the international manner of YYYYMMDD to avoid cross-border confusion. Note that other segments are available; however, these are the most likely to be encountered in the imaging informatics profession. A full list can be found in the HL7 specification documents and are regularly updated as uses evolve.

Message Types

Within the message header, the type of message is defined. With over 50 message types to choose from, those most commonly observed are given in *Table 9.2*.

As part of the message type, ADT (admit, discharge, or transfer) is an instruction to do something (the task the A0x code relates to). As HL7 messaging operates on a 'read-back' confirmation basis (similar

Table 9.2 Common HL7 message types

Prefix	Value	Description
ADT *or* ACK	A01	Admit a patient/visit notification
ADT *or* ACK	A02	Transfer a patient
ADT *or* ACK	A03	Discharge a patient/end this visit
ADT *or* ACK	A04	Register a patient
ADT *or* ACK	A05	Pre-admit a patient
ADT *or* ACK	A06	Change an O/P to an I/P
ADT *or* ACK	A08	Update patient information/record
ADT *or* ACK	A11	Cancel admission of patient
ADT *or* ACK	A12	Cancel transfer of patient
ADT *or* ACK	A13	Cancel discharge of patient
ADT *or* ACK	A18	Merge patient information/record

ACK, acknowledging response; ADT, admit, discharge, or transfer; HL7, health level 7.

to air traffic control instructions to pilots), the prefix of ADT or ACK is appended depending on whether it is the original instruction from the requesting system, or the acknowledging response from the receiving system. For example, a message sent from a MPI to RIS with an ADT-A04 is instructing the RIS to register a patient (with details supplied in the later PID segment of the same message); RIS completes the action requested and replies with an identical message, except replacing with an acknowledgement value in the message header: ACK-A04. This confirms the message has been received correctly, rather than corrupted in transfer.

IHE

The IHE initiative exists to utilise existing standards and processes to better facilitate sharing of data between healthcare IT systems. In order to do this, IHE provides a number of integration profiles; these profiles take an example use-case and describe how to best apply existing standards in order to prevent future difficulties with interoperability.

IHE as a group also organises annual events known as 'connectathons' where vendors meet to test interoperability with each other's systems (both software and hardware), particularly focussing on HL7 and DICOM compatibility, ensuring there are fewer chances of integration issues in clinical departments.

FHIR

Pronounced 'Fire', Fast Healthcare Interoperability Resources (FHIR) is being developed as a new add-on set of resources by the HL7 International Organisation to address some of the inflexibilities the traditional HL7 standards possess by utilising newer programming methodologies and web-based coding languages (HTML, cascading style sheets, etc.). Its development has been encouraged by the continuing move to digitisation of all types of health records, in their many forms, locations, and formats, which current standards struggle to unite cohesively.

CHAPTER 10

DATA SHARING AND TELERADIOLOGY

At their most basic, digital radiological studies are simply computer files, which can be transmitted around in any suitable manner. In today's mobile society, with years of digital images available and an emphasis on collaborative care, the ability to move patient data around efficiently and securely but rapidly is an important one. Radiology departments generate two main forms of data requiring movement – text and imaging (picture) files. Text, primarily in the form of study reports, is relatively simple to move around with many established methods; however, owing to their size and nature of viewing, images present more of a challenge. Competition within the UK has increased the number of vendors supplying institutions with PACS, and has left a situation where there is no central index of images, making sharing more technically complex. Coupled with the lack of a central index, another major limitation on simple sharing is interoperability; some PACS suppliers have been slow to move towards utilising standards and methods that would allow relatively simple interconnections between each other's systems, as obviously this has commercial considerations.

History of Radiological Image Sharing

The historic origins of radiological data sharing stem from the simple physical forwarding of the fragile glass photographic plates in the early parts of the 20th century, through to the use of copy films, to laser film prints, to CDs, and then towards digital duplication of electronic data files.

Some of these early methods suffered from degradations or drawbacks, meaning the benefits of attempting to share the data had to be considered carefully. Some of these drawbacks included the risk of physical damage (glass plates), generational loss (dark-room copied films), and print medium scaling defects (laser film). In addition, CDs, DVDs, and removable media can be lost, stolen, or intercepted and are not easily auditable from end-to-end. Newer transfer methods mitigate these risks – digital copies do not degrade on a per copy basis, and can be transmitted electronically, almost instantaneously and with full accountability, removing the risk of damaging or losing the 'only copy' while in transit. The practice of creating CDs for transfer continued well into the 2010s. However, as the national intra-NHS N3 network became faster, with more hospitals establishing connections and the shift in clinical practice towards moving patients onwards for specialist care, better, faster, and more secure techniques were required. Now, with the advent of numerous electronic transfer methods available via the internet or the N3 network, it is possible to transfer imaging without the need to create physical copies at all.

Methods of Sharing Radiological Images

The primary methods utilised by NHS hospitals to move images between otherwise unconnected sites within the UK are:

- Electronically via 3rd party software or portals (the Image Exchange Portal [IEP] being the de-facto system in use within the UK).
- Electronically via regional solutions (where a PACS provider connects their own systems together in a proprietary manner).
- Physically via offline media: CD/DVD/Blu-Ray/USB/HDD.
- Physically: printed A4 sheets.
- Electronically: JPEGs via email or other.

- Physically: film or other hard copy.
- Electronically via XDS (where multiple PACS providers utilise standards and initiatives to connect in a non-proprietary manner).
- Electronically: NHS Secure File Transfer service.

Reasons for Sharing Radiological Data

The most common reasons for transfer are varied:

- Clinical opinion (referral/relocation of patient unlikely).
- Clinical opinion (referral/relocation likely).
- Reporting.
- Contractual (routine outsourcing of certain types of exams, such as CT/MRI brain, perhaps using the Any Qualified Provider [AQP] services, or those provided on relocatable 'vans').
- Shared MDT meetings.
- Referred/standard referral (without opinion owing to set patient pathways).
- Clinical collaboration with specialist colleagues (a 'second opinion').
- Teaching.
- Contractual (on-call or out-of-hours reasons): requested by a radiologist (in contemplation of another action – with no specific reason at present, but gets the transfer process underway).

Other, less common, reasons for image sharing include sending images for 3D printing or templating (e.g. for customised aortic stents), feedback for those on clinical trials co-ordinated typically from America, health tourism (overseas patients travelling to the UK for paid treatment unavailable in their home country), and private patients seeking copies to obtain multiple opinions or move between providers.

Electronic Sharing Methods

Numerous electronic transfer methods are now available via the internet or the intra-NHS (N3) network, making it possible to target recipients and track progress without the historic use of creating hard copies, CDs or DVDs with a 'signed-for' courier.

Networked image sharing can be one of three broad types – mailbox, cloud, or direct (**Figs 10.1–10.3**).

- Mailbox-based methods allow an upload into a specific virtual mailbox, for an entire healthcare institution, a service group, or a specific clinician.
- Cloud-based services provide an off-site storage of imaging data and allow for the images to be exchanged in a portal or other web-based application.
- The approach taken for direct sharing varies and can involve creating a remote connection to a PACS or by utilising new technical architectures, such as XDS-I. An example of a peer-to-peer (point-to-point) connection is below, but different vendors apply different levels of complexity to the process.

Many currently used electronic sharing methods have a significant drawback – they commonly create copies of imaging, duplicating the files with no automated update link back to the original source. A lack of synchronisation creates difficulties in being sure that the copies remain the most current and complete record for the patient after receipt. Images received electronically should be considered 'valid' only at the time of transfer, with decreasing confidence in reliability as time passes thereafter. Owing to this, it is therefore good practice to avoid routinely storing all electronically received copies permanently

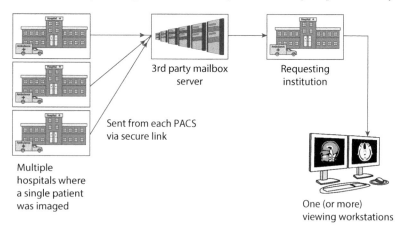

3rd party mailbox server

Requesting institution

Sent from each PACS via secure link

Multiple hospitals where a single patient was imaged

One (or more) viewing workstations

Fig. 10.1 Mailbox sharing. (PACS, picture archiving and communication system.)

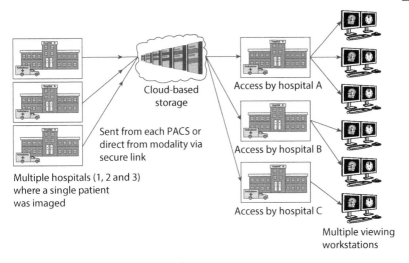

Fig. 10.2 Cloud sharing. (PACS, picture archiving and communication system.)

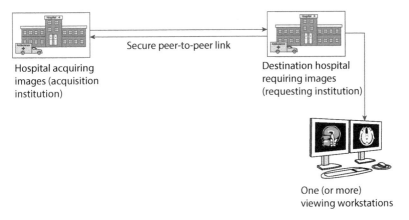

Fig. 10.3 Direct sharing.

(perhaps a 14-day rule should be used), and to avoid, as much as possible, the temptation to forward on a copy of the copy to another site (the third site should instead revert to the originating institution to obtain up-to-date records in case any changes have occurred in the intervening period since the original transfer). This allows for accurate record keeping at the originating institution and the possibility of alerting known recipients if a patient misidentification or other issue with the images is later identified, plus balances the legal risks over who is actually responsible for any 'error' introduced into the process. Prior to carrying out any procedure, it remains the responsibility of the recipient site to check that images are still complete and current before relying upon them for treatment purposes; this may require re-requesting images from the originating institution if necessary.

The National Image Exchange Portal

Familiar to many, the National Image Exchange Portal (IEP) is used by all NHS Acute Trusts and all major private healthcare institutions within England and Northern Ireland, as well as extensively across Scotland and Wales. The IEP is by far the most commonly used method of transferring radiological images outside of regional sharing hubs within the UK. It utilises the mailbox design to transfer tens of thousands of images and reports daily, with organisations using the service only requiring one connection into their PACS. Data sent in and out are encrypted and transferred either via the private intra-NHS N3 network or via the general internet, as necessary. Access to the service is via a web-based portal used to both request and transfer the images, with management of the system being by local PACS Managers.

In order to reduce the number of duplicate images in the country and risk associated with these, a number of institutions have begun also introducing an extension based on the XDS standard known as IEP Connect & Share. This system is still in its infancy, but appears to present the closest opportunity towards creation of a single image index (and potentially repository) possible so far.

Regional Sharing

Where a single PACS vendor (or a combination of vendors working in partnership) has multiple installations, they may offer to link these together utilising an internal proprietary sharing solution, typically providing neighbouring sites access to each other's systems as if they were one. This is currently found in Northern Ireland (one group), Scotland (another group), Wales, and clusters in England, including the Liverpool & Mersey region, Southampton, Hampshire, and Isle of Wight plus several others on a smaller scale.

North-West PACS Portal

This portal, initially designed and developed by a radiologist of the Christie NHS Foundation Trust, allows users of multiple different PACS systems (even different vendors) access to each other's systems by acting as an intermediary. It is widely used in the region it was originally introduced into and has won multiple awards for solving the interoperability problem around image sharing at a time when image sharing was treated as mainly a physical process.

Teleradiology

Simplified, this is where images are acquired in one location, stored on a single PACS, but reported from a different physical location (but still onto the same PACS/RIS) without the images being copied. It is commonplace in four main circumstances:

1 Delivery of speciality coverage of large areas, e.g. Scotland, where one or more specialist reporting staff cover more than one hospital (because there is insufficient demand to dedicate their time to one location).

2 Where equipment is available to acquire images, but a speciality reporting post is temporarily vacant.

3 Outsourcing purposes: commonly where 'backlog' reporting is required to help reduce the number of outstanding unreported cases, or overnight cover is required by reporting staff utilising 'follow-the-sun' principles, e.g. in Australia.

4 Home-based reporting: to allow reporting staff primarily based in the acquiring institution to report from home overnight (on-call), or carry out ad-hoc additional reporting sessions (post retirement etc.).

QA AND MEDICAL PHYSICS CONSIDERATIONS

QA throughout Radiology departments is commonplace – for modalities utilising ionising radiation, tasks such as checking X-ray tube output, exposure duration plus collimation/beam accuracy, together with performing test studies on contrast phantoms are routine. In modalities utilising non-ionising radiation, similar tests are carried out, but are tailored to the imaging parameters involved. The hardware, software, and applications underpinning the imaging informatics speciality also require similar attention to ensure that images remain available and accessible when needed. The Institute of Physics and Engineering in Medicine (IPEM) reports detail good practices in this area, with common QA actions involving regular considerations in the areas described below.

Display Monitors

The initial choice of display monitors for both reporting workstations and general-use PCs is critical. Image display monitors for the purposes of viewing radiological imaging are broken down into two main types:

1 Diagnostic display monitors (primary displays) (**Fig. 11.1**) are used to view imaging to determine treatment or patient pathway progression prior to a report being issued – this can be, for instance, the case of

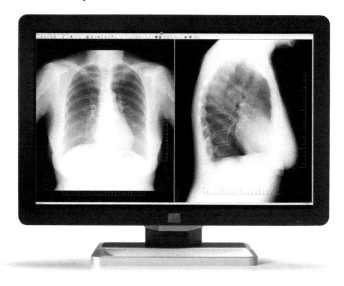

Fig. 11.1 An example of a diagnostic display.

clinicians viewing an image in A&E to determine the patient's condition, or for reporting staff on reporting workstations to view images and generate a report. They are expensive, ranging from £2,000 to £40,000 per screen depending on quality and task (displays designed for the review of breast imaging are at the higher end of the cost spectrum), and are usually purchased in matched pairs for ergonomic reasons. These will additionally require a specialist high-end graphics card in the attached workstation, pushing the package price at the upper end towards £100,000.

2 Review monitors (secondary displays) (**Fig. 11.2**) are used when a report has already been issued, and the monitor is purely being used in conjunction with an officially issued interpretation (the report) for guidance. These monitors range from £1,000 to £10,000 for a pair of screens with suitable graphics card.

The required sizing of monitors is constantly debated, with medical imaging screens being measured in megapixels (MP) – millions of pixels – rather than the traditional inch or pixel dimensions common

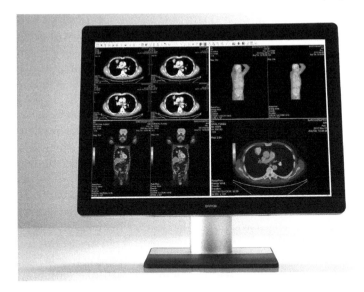

Fig. 11.2 An example of a review monitor.

with televisions and projectors. In the current environments, 6 MP colour monitors are commonly offered for sale as diagnostic displays, with 1 MP or 2 MP colour monitors offered as review screens.

While most reporting workstations within a Radiology department will have diagnostic displays attached, considerations must be given to areas dependent on viewing images immediately after imaging without the benefit of a report. These areas should also ideally be provided with diagnostic displays, with other high-traffic areas, such as clinics or ward-round stations, being provided with at least one (slightly lesser quality) review monitor. Remember, much reporting is also carried out by suitably trained radiographers, nurse practitioners, speech and language therapists, and general clinicians: plus 'red dot' systems, by general radiographers – these professionals may not have easy access to radiology reporting rooms and this will need consideration. Further inexpensive monitors of the generic 'domestic' type, perhaps for viewing RIS textual data or general internet usage, are not included in the above. Obviously all areas would be best served by diagnostic screens, but cost is a prohibitive factor in fulfilling this.

Ongoing maintenance of primary and secondary displays is of the utmost importance. With electronic acquisition, distribution, and display of images now being standard, modern day healthcare institutions are heavily dependent on properly functioning display devices. Both the pixels and backlights within flat-panel monitors degrade or fail with age (and use) and should be regularly checked. Tests on review monitors can be as simple as reviewing a set of images with various test patterns and recording the results; for diagnostic displays the tests must be more comprehensive, with calibration to a DICOM response curve being carried out (if not built in and automated) utilising a 'puck' test device and software at least annually. Many diagnostic monitors are now designed to carry out basic daily self-tests, reporting back to a piece of monitoring software located on a server within the healthcare institution in order to supplement the more comprehensive medical physics testing and provide faster alerting to monitors out of calibration. In addition, web-based image viewing software can include a display suitability test (typically asking the viewer to enter characters buried in contrast test image).

Basic day-to-day maintenance of all monitor types also includes careful cleaning (the sometimes 'interactive' nature of reporting generates finger marks on screens, with grease from these marks being found to obscure portions of images or even pathologies on occasion). Cleaning with the correct solutions is of the utmost importance, as scratching of the surface of monitors or damage to the evenness of the anti-glare or anti-reflection coatings causes typically irreparable damage.

Reporting Environment

The technology around monitors is changing rapidly. Owing to the move from cold cathode fluorescent lamp (CCFL) to light-emitting diode (LED) backlights (LED being more powerful, but held to a moderate brightness level using user-configurable software and integrated photometric sensors), a completely darkened room is no longer necessary for reporting in, rather only comfortable but even lighting is required. Light levels in reporting locations therefore need to be reassessed as new monitors are purchased.

The physical surroundings and environment in healthcare institutions also change over time – not only can window coverings change and ceiling lights be updated as fashion and décor dictate, but also portable lights around display devices can be altered, surfaces become more highly reflective, walls painted more brightly, and windows uncovered. This is especially noticeable in ward or trauma areas, which may not consider the requirements for diagnostic or review displays in their refurbishment plans. The suitability of viewing locations should therefore be assessed as required, taking note of advice from medical physics personnel.

Reporting areas internal to a Radiology department can either be communal spaces in the form of a shared large custom designed 'reporting room', or simply a collection of individual offices, each with one or more reporting workstations located within them. Shared communal reporting rooms have the advantage that it becomes an easier task to locate traditionally elusive reporting staff, particularly of less-common specialities, but the environment within these can quickly become disruptive and noisy if access is not strictly controlled. General tidiness of shared rooms also suffers in the same way as any shared space in the workplace with clutter, unwashed cups, and the ubiquitous (and often outdated) laminated A4 sheets seen to begin taking over entire stretches of wall space in a similar manner to moss propagating over a stone wall.

The ideal reporting environment consists of the correct combination of the following main physical parameters:

- Temperature.
- Lighting.
- Sound levels.
- Distractions.
- Comfort and facilities.

When designing a reporting environment or undertaking a refurbishment of a Radiology department, consideration should be given to the input of psychological professionals, in order to maximise the benefits of human factors on workplace environments (in much the same way as consulting on waiting room design to help increase patient satisfaction and compliance).

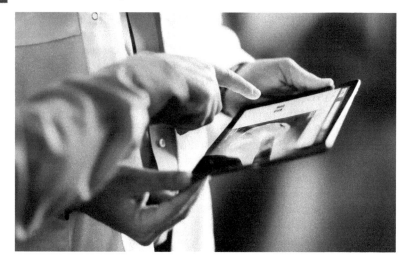

Fig. 11.3 Greater utilisation of tablet devices for viewing PACS images on wards and clinics.

Designing image viewing areas on wards or in A&E departments is generally outside of the influence of imaging informatics professionals, but every attempt should be made to replicate similar suggestions for those areas upon redesign: including the provision of dedicated purpose-designed 'hot' (live) reporting areas.

A major challenge for QA purposes comes from the modern availability of report accessibility. Many PACS now offer web-based access for home reporting, and with clinicians now regularly being able to access images on handheld and tablet devices (**Fig. 11.3**), plus reporting staff at remote locations, such as from home on laptops, maintaining an optimum reporting environment in less controllable circumstances is one of the most difficult tasks of running a successful informatics service in imaging.

Staff

A classic 'oversight' when designing QA protocols for informatics equipment is to overlook routine eye testing for reporting staff. Within the UK, all staff utilising a VDU are required to be afforded eye tests, paid for by their employer (or in Scotland eye tests remain free for all), and staff should be encouraged to utilise these at least annually. This reduces the likelihood of having an optimal monitor set-up and reporting/viewing environment, but defective eyesight reducing the quality actually seen.

Business Continuity

For many of the above tasks, medical physics involvement is crucial; however, there are other considerations relating to QA of the actual software processes. One of these is preparing for the possibility of component degradation or unexpected outages and identifying which processes are critical and which would not place patients at increased risk if they failed unexpectedly.

These potential failures must be matched against local clinical impact, e.g. if a monitor is found to be faulty this may not sound (or be treated) as serious to a general non-clinical IT department call handler. If, however, this monitor was the sole device for viewing images in a sterile zone (such as in theatres) or in a restricted area (such as request viewing in nuclear medicine isotope preparation rooms) it would require different prioritisation. Likewise, if a printer failed this may not be assessed as critical; however, if this printer is the output for hardcopy log files from a legacy server, it may not be long before buffers (temporary storages) fill up and the server stops processing new transactions – a previously common problem in the banking industry, or for payroll departments.

A recent concern raised by current technological developments with shifts towards off-premises storage of medical imaging in cloud-based storage is the consideration that cloud-based providers can just 'shut-up-shop' if the service is not generating enough income. One of the final Google Health developer blog entries has a thinly veiled reference to commercial considerations in relation to closure of the Google Health Cloud, with just 12 months allowed for users to migrate data to another platform.

Taking both on-site and off-site processes into consideration, testing of the end-to-end workflow (from request to dispatch of report) with dummy data at routine intervals is wise and prudent practice given the number of interconnections and complexities that exist in a modern informatics implementation. This should occur along with documenting the possible alternatives to accomplishing each step should a component fail (e.g. entering scheduling data into an EPR or other system should the RIS 'calendar' function become unavailable owing to a fault). Reverting to a paper-based system (perhaps for requesting imaging when an OCS interface into RIS fails) is a common contingency. Having these alternative plans available and tested ensures that the 'business' of healthcare provision can continue uninterrupted in exigent circumstances (albeit sometimes in a slower and clunkier manner!).

Disaster Recovery

Leading from business continuity planning, rehearsing or practising a disaster recovery (DR) scenario also forms part of a well-designed QA programme. All too often, imaging informatics personnel forget that disasters can occur and are not prepared for them – this places unnecessarily high burdens on other parts of the healthcare institution as the standard routines staff follow are unavailable. Creating a basic DR strategy is as simple as drafting a set of steps that should be followed should a component of the service fail in order to mitigate or reduce disruption (e.g. if the PACS archive fails or if network services are lost). Ideally, these should be practised.

Common business continuity and disaster recovery plans include:

- PACS failure (unable to view images).
- PACS failure (full/unable to store images).
- PACS failure (image or database loss).
- Cyber-attack response and mitigation.
- Modality worklist failure.
- Power loss in department.
- RIS failure (scheduling and exam data unavailable/lost).
- OCS to RIS interface failure (request data unavailable).
- RIS to EPR interface failure (report data unavailable).
- Network failure (images cannot be transmitted to PACS).
- Hardware failures (reporting workstations unavailable).
- Recovery from physical damage to the server room (data or hardware loss caused by fire, flood, physical attack, or software attack/ virus/malware).

Other system administrators will create plans for loss of systems under their remit (OCS, EPR) and should be consulted to craft a robust enterprise-wide strategy.

Image Acquisition Faults

As with historic film and chemical processes, modern digital acquisition methods suffer from some common and not so common faults. These can give characteristic appearances on the resultant imaging or errors, the most frequent of which should be either mitigated against, or educated for, in order to reduce their impact. These faults present themselves in different ways for different modalities and are studied in many external publications: for examples of CR or DDR faults, see *Clark's Positioning in Radiography*, 13th edition, page 38.

Testing

Another of the most frequently unappreciated tasks of local informatics support teams is testing prior to clinical use of a new or upgraded system. Local testing should deliver a structured, clear, and disciplined investigation into the behaviour of a new or modified system and should not be left to the software supplier to carry out (after all, they will not be using the system to treat their patients). Good test regimens should report their findings by cross-reference to agreed requirements, declare any working assumptions, and feed back on any unintended consequences encountered. Without testing there may be adverse effects to people, patient safety, and organisations from a business point of view (either time, money, confidence, or reputational damage in this context).

The three main considerations for software testing, which can also be adopted for hardware, are:
- A test plan.
- Preparation.
- Test execution.

A Test Plan

A test plan should be created, with a structure including:
- Objectives (purpose).
- Scope for what will be included and excluded.
- Interface specifications.
- Assumptions of other systems that will be tested simultaneously.
- Traceability to requirements (via the contract/schedule of work/ specification).

- Testing stages (in sequential order):
    - proof of concept (especially if new system);
    - unit;
    - system;
    - system integration testing;
    - user acceptance testing (UAT);
    - data migration (if relevant);
    - production acceptance testing (if needed).

Preparation

Preparation is key before the testing starts, in the form of a test readiness review after the supplier has indicated they are ready to deploy (formally passed the 'test entry gate'). This should include:

- Handover documentation.
- Test summary report.
- Plan that the deploying department will have written or had input into.
- Test scripts that provide the detailed steps of each test and the expected result of each.
- Schedules and timelines.
- Resources for relevant stages to include:
    - test domain, i.e. controlled environment that changes can be made on, then tested before and after the system is deployed;
    - necessary equipment and accounts and configuration that will replicate the live environment;
    - staff required to test.

Test Execution

Test execution includes:

- Sources of test data, such as test patients, images, or simulators.
- Test evidence/test scripts to include reference documentation, patient names, ID, workflow identifiers, stage, steps required, dates, tester name.
- Progress reports, containing metrics of outstanding issues and progress through the cycles (typically in the form of a spreadsheet, allowing tracking and updates to be entered as the testing progresses).

- Recording of results – the expected steps should match actual results:

  – passes need to be recorded (with evidence);

  – any unexpected results can be managed by recording the information, from the test evidence via screenshots or utilising the Microsoft Windows Problem Step Recorder (available in Windows 7 and above), plus adding an indicative severity level along with the output message.

- Frequent reviews during testing need to be conducted daily as 'wash up' calls at specific times, reviewing new issues, and closing existing ones.

- If working in an environment where remedies to defects are to be applied and re-tested, this must be done in a controlled manner – consideration towards re-testing previously passed tests should be considered to ensure they remain unaffected by the newest changes.

CHAPTER 12

CLINICIANS' INFORMATION NEEDS: A CLINICIAN'S PERSPECTIVE

Clinicians utilise radiological data for many different purposes, the most common being:

■ For diagnosis (patient present, e.g. in clinic).
■ For diagnosis (patient not present, e.g. on wards).
■ During preparation/presentation in an MDT meeting (**Fig. 12.1**).
■ For teaching.
■ To assist a colleague (have 'a quick look').
■ Social media/self-interest purposes.

Modern medical care aims to deliver effective healthcare in a timely fashion while maintaining high levels of patient satisfaction. Good performance in the delivery of this service is dependent upon accurate diagnosis, use of diagnostic tools such as imaging, appropriate treatment, and the patient's perceived experience through the healthcare system – the 'patient's journey'. Medical imaging coupled with complimentary software systems plays a major role in accurate diagnosis of medical and surgical conditions, guides interventional and surgical

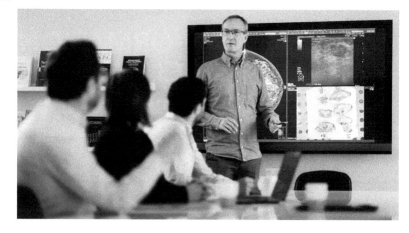

Fig. 12.1 Case presentation at a multidisciplinary team meeting.

treatment, and enables the clinician to empower the patient in the decision-making process. Greater education and discussion allows our patients to make more informed decisions regarding their own treatment. By managing patient expectations we can improve patient compliance and satisfaction, and overall provide better patient care. In this chapter the role of the radiographer and radiologist as 'producers', and the role of the clinician and patient as 'consumers' will be outlined from an orthopaedic surgeon's perspective: giving an overview of how the information seeking behaviour of clinicians has changed with time, and providing insight into how best radiographers can support 'consumers' in the future.

The Patient Journey: Radiographers as Producers, Clinicians as Consumers

Growing emphasis has been placed on the satisfaction associated with the 'patient journey' as a quality indicator in modern healthcare trusts. The journey, as shown in *Table 12.1*, begins when a patient presents to the service by being either electively referred by their GP, from other healthcare professionals, or acutely through A&E. A clinician

Table 12.1 Components of a satisfactory patient consultation

	Stage 1	Adequate history
+	Stage 2	Diagnostics: imaging (CR/DDR, US, CT, MR, etc.) + pathology + haematology…
+	Stage 3	Examination
+	Stage 4	Patient education (including treatment)
=	Outcome	Patient satisfaction and compliance with treatment

CR/DDR, computed radiography/direct digital radiography; CT, computed tomography; MR, magnetic resonance; US, ultrasound.

(a consumer of radiological services) will attempt to take a detailed history and usually examine the patient. As consumers, clinicians will extract the data relevant to any radiological request to formulate a working diagnosis to explain the patient's symptoms. This diagnosis is either confirmed or refuted by various basic investigations and occasionally supplemented by more advanced investigations. Having a widely connected EPR, with fast access to the patient's medical history, saves time and questioning of the patient (who indeed may be unable to recall, or even answer, at the time of presentation).

Treatment is commenced, and either continues in the community or the patient is admitted to hospital for possible further investigations and follow-up. Clinicians rely on the producers (the Radiology department for imaging) to provide prompt, accurate, and easily accessible services, allowing the patients to be managed correctly (**Fig.12.2**).

The patient's journey can be affected in many ways, both positively and negatively. Streamlined services and 'one stop clinics', such as breast clinics, where all component services are available one after another on the same day improve efficiency, patient satisfaction, and allow prompt medical treatment. Additionally, nationwide '2-week wait' cancer pathway referrals are treated with urgency from the first clinician appointment to imaging completion. These national targets are improving access to prompt treatment by prioritising patients who may otherwise inadvertently just become another number in today's busy hospitals. As patient consumption of healthcare services increases, we are likely to see patient journeys being negatively impacted on while struggling to meet demand.

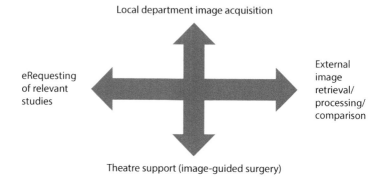

Fig. 12.2 Interaction between consumers (clinicians) and producers.

To combat this, streamlining services are required. The transition from paper medical records to an electronic format is currently ongoing across the UK and serves to make the process of assimilating information regarding a patient and their past medical history more accessible, complete, and reliably traceable. The ease of availability in turn aids the clinician formulating a working diagnosis, and in planning future treatment or surgery. It has been shown that when electronic medical records are available to radiologists the reporting quality is improved, as the original clinical information on radiological request forms is often inadequate (the bare minimum to allow a request to be 'accepted' by a radiographer). Problems arise when crucial results or documents are not uploaded onto the system in a timely manner, or when the patient has undergone medical or surgical treatment at a different healthcare institution and consequently there are no records to corroborate the patient's story. In such cases, the records are incomplete and this can lead to a clinical risk, delayed treatment, or duplicating investigations (including re-irradiation in radiology).

Patients have different expectations of healthcare, particularly as they compare to current domestic technologies available to them. They not only expect that their medical notes are available freely between their GP and their local hospital, but also between different hospitals. Understandably, patients are often frustrated when their medical notes, imaging, or discharge letters are not routinely available between sites, and struggle to understand why this is. This often contributes to a delay in investigation or treatment, creating potential difficulties with planning surgical interventions at different hospital locations, as well as leading to wasted hospital visits as decisions may not be confirmed until that information later becomes available. Not only is this inconvenient for the patient, but also it delays provision of services to other patients while the 'problem' is resolved, potentially impacting on a number of individual patient journeys. This highlights the key role of the 'producers' and the importance of ensuring results and information are uploaded onto the electronic systems swiftly and accurately. Where this is not done it can have a direct impact on the 'consumers' with potential delays in diagnosis and treatment impacting on both clinicians and patients.

The investigative process in healthcare involves clinicians acting as consumers, and radiographers acting as producers of various imaging modalities, to help them provide effective healthcare. The information seeking behaviours of clinicians is in many ways aligned with the expectations placed upon them by current social demands and the evolving patient profile. Modern society places higher demands on the systems designed to provide a service, both in the volume of patients consuming services, and an individual's expectations of what these services can provide to them, both medically and socially.

Speed and convenience are at the forefront of what is considered efficient in today's 'snowflake' generation 24/7 attitude. Effective and efficient care is expected to be delivered in a timely fashion. These timescales are far removed from what was once previously considered acceptable by society, where waiting lists for elective surgery were over 1 year. This has led to the dawn of a new era of '7 day elective services' to accommodate the increasing demand and availability of services. The cultural shift seen in recent years results in an ever growing interdependence between clinicians and radiographers to enable both high quality care and targets to be met. As a result of these wider changes to society, to some extent medicine is now practised in a defensive manner as the chances of being sued for a missed diagnosis, or repercussions from a delay in starting treatment are far increased, further increasing demand on services.

The past decade has also seen a substantial growth in complex radiological interventions and in many cases, such as cardiology, patient outcomes are dependent upon these services being readily available. The development of interventional radiology, e.g. in terms of vascular angioplasty, has reduced the demand on the surgical speciality by treating these patients awake and as day cases, improving patient satisfaction. However interventional radiology is not universally available throughout NHS Trusts, leading to variation in the skillset provided to patients geographically. This in itself can lead to problems, deskilling surgeons in some specialities in both clinical decision making and technical skills where interventional radiology is expanding, as well as exposing patients to more invasive procedures in areas where interventional radiology is not available.

Traditional Medical Practice

In the 'good old days' medicine was practiced in a very didactic and authoritative manner. The patient hung on their clinician's every word and there was very little (if any) discussion or challenge on the treatment options available. The decision-making process fell solely to the hands of the clinician and the patient was expected to comply without question. The process of 'diagnosis' involved the use of meticulous clinical examination skills, blood tests, and basic imaging data, such as plain radiographs, presented in the form of acetate films that were viewed on a light box. The radiographers were expected to produce these films and there was little in the way of dialogue between the producer and the consumer except via the sections on the request card. Traditional imaging requests were paper based and the responsibility of the junior doctor on the team. Often, this doctor and the patient had little understanding of the indication to request the test; however, all requests would need discussion between the junior doctor and a radiologist or radiographer. There was a huge administrative burden when handling these paper requests with no way of reliably tracking requests or their progress, and often they would be lost, delayed, and frequently this even resulted in duplicated requests. Images were acquired as physical films and again there were inefficiencies in the handling and storage of such images. The junior doctor was expected to assimilate all these films from the patient notes for the purpose of the daily morning departmental meeting and then return them after the meeting ended. The number of steps involved in simply handling these films would often lead to misplaced or lost films, even when disregarding the process inefficiencies in the Radiology department itself. Another limitation associated with such acquisition was the inability to manipulate these images for better viewing and the inability to quickly share the images if an expert opinion was sought from the consultant at home, or from other departments or hospitals. Similarly, traditional imaging reports were also paper based and left in the requesting clinician's pigeon-hole for checking. This slow process was fraught with problems, such as lost or untraceable reports and late notification of critical findings, all negatively impacting on the patient journey and the quality and pace of the service provided. To clinicians, the old physical films did, however, have some benefits as the clinician was not tethered to a viewing terminal and therefore consultations had the potential to be more patient focused as images could be viewed with the patient at the bedside by holding the images up to a ceiling light or window.

Modern Medical Practice

From the early 2000s there have been many progressions in medicine, and radiography is no exception to this. This has directly impacted on the patient journey and alters the interaction between radiographers as producers and clinicians as consumers. Modern health provision is heavily weighted towards evidence-based clinical practice to provide the best possible care to our patients, coupled with an awareness to adhere to nationally imposed targets that have financial implications for the hospital. Advances in imaging modalities have allowed more accurate diagnosis than before and, therefore, the potential for earlier or more specific treatment. The current healthcare system faces the challenge of managing larger volumes of patients with an ageing population, with financial penalties enforced if care is not provided within a timely fashion. Current medical practice has evolved into a more patient-centred approach where consultations are expected to be a discussion of options so that the patient can make an informed decision regarding the treatment they receive. Patient education and autonomy forms the keystone of any successful treatment plan and improves patient compliance. Imaging plays a pivotal role, providing 'evidence' to the patient, enabling quick and accurate diagnoses to be made in many conditions, and we have seen an evolution of the processes involved in acquiring these images.

Modern requests are IT based and often the responsibility of the senior clinician who has reviewed the patient and been involved in the discussion, rather than handed down to a junior as before. Electronic requests are governed by individual log-in accounts and are easily tracked to monitor progression and avoid duplication. Requests are often triaged on the same day and appointment allocation is also IT based. This transition has reduced the administrative burden and the process is less time-consuming for the clinician; it allows the provision of better clinical information to justify the imaging, and provides better legibility of the request. Radiology departments can also customise additional questions to be answered, saving time if, for example, creatinine levels are required before authorisation of a study.

Modern technology has also allowed imaging to be acquired and viewed in a digital format – a stark contrast from the traditional physical films. In the UK, these images can be viewed on most computer terminals and so can 'follow the clinician' so long as there is a workstation nearby. Image retrieval is a logged action and therefore this system also complies with good governance principles, which states that a clinician is only justified in accessing information regarding a patient whose care they are involved with. The various advantages and disadvantages of digital imaging from a general clinician's perspective are listed in *Table 12.2*.

Table 12.2 Key advantages and disadvantages of the transition from analogue to digital images

Advantages of digital imaging	Disadvantages of digital imaging
Easier storage and handling	Tethering to fixed viewing stations
Images can be manipulated	Slow processing of large volumes of data
Allows templating for surgical planning	Potential for hardware failure
Allows image sharing	Potential for software failure
Better display options for MDT meetings	Training requirements
Viewing history is logged to comply with clinical governance requirements	Access (account/password) issues

MDT, multidisciplinary team.

The representation of digital images on screens with well-adapted specifications provides a medium for accurate diagnosis, with images that can be manipulated and can be more readily shared between teams and hospitals. The transition from analogue to digital also allows easier storage, although a common drawback observed across the country is longer loading times in more remote wards when the IT network is inundated. Modern reporting systems are much more efficient and provide better guidance than traditional paper and tape cassette recorder methodologies; however, many systems still lack a fluid feedback channel between the requesting clinician and the reporting clinician (who may be a reporting radiographer, radiologist, nurse, AHP, or indeed a chest clinician, etc.). Another drawback in the move towards a paperless imaging process is the perceived less judicious requesting of images when some might regard certain images as unnecessary. Indeed, time-pressured clinical staff may feel more easily persuaded into requesting additional imaging if the access to the services is easier and smoother than with historic paper and legwork to the Radiology department (carrying down the request forms).

Despite occasional long loading times when the network is at capacity, the shift of medical imaging from analogue to digital format has allowed more efficient image processing, speeding up their availability to clinicians. Digital images are viewed and manipulated on software programs, which increases the scope for sharing images between departments and Trusts with relative ease. The interpretation of these images is dependent upon the availability of workstations or monitors that are specifically designed for viewing medical images. However, the main limitation at present is that clinicians remain tethered to these workstations rather than being able to involve the patient in the 'viewing' and 'thinking' processes over their care. Some UK sites utilise 'workstations-on-wheels' – portable workstations that can be wheeled to the bedside; however, the use of high-resolution tablets is now beginning to take place and may prove to resolve this tethering issue in the future. The core limiting factors to these more mobile methods is the availability of reliable secure wireless network access points within hospitals to load the images: a problem that is difficult to solve in older, more densely built hospital sites as was traditional in the UK, as well as considerations around viewing environment suitability.

Patient's Evolving Consumer Profile

Many consultant-level staff began their medical school training in a culture where diagnosis was almost entirely based on taking a detailed and relevant history corroborated with a good clinical examination. There was little reliance on medical imaging and accessibility to these modalities was sparse. One would wait for weeks for an MRI or CT scan. The development of new imaging modalities, coupled with improved imaging hardware and software, has improved accurate diagnoses. However, it is not without its own problems, as it also increases the chances of incidental findings: that may or may not be significant or relevant to the patient and may result in further investigation and invasive tests.

Clinicians have since learned that clinical signs only provide part of the picture and consequently have become increasingly reliant on imaging to make an accurate diagnosis. Therefore as a consumer, clinicians have changed. Clinicians have become much more demanding of these services and resources as they become increasingly reliant upon them to diagnose, treat, and monitor patients' progress. Clinicians want and need to practise medicine with seamless technological integration and want answers quickly. The use of mobile devices facilitates bedside patient education and both formal and informal multidisciplinary discussion of patients to draw upon the wealth of experience available to clinicians within the hospital setting.

Evolving Patient Profile

Social gentrification has bred a growing desire to be informed and autonomous. Patient education and autonomy form the keystone of any successful treatment plan and improves patient compliance. Patients now frequently use the internet as a source of medical education – this information is brought to the consultation and forms part of the 'informed' discussion regarding treatment. Patient expectations have changed: patients raise questions based on what they have read and expect an immediate answer. Patients also expect to be involved in the decision-making process, and expect quick and efficient service. Home-based technology has rapidly advanced in the last decade, not only in the development of new technologies but also the availability of these technologies to the public as prices become more reasonable. Patients no longer see colour television as a luxury; they are watching 4K ultra-high definition or 3D television on a daily basis. They are no longer dialling up to join the internet, but downloading films on their mobile phone on their commute to work. It is understandable that they would expect that this level of technology would be available in healthcare services if it is available on the high street at a reasonable price.

The word 'service' defines the modern provision of healthcare. We provide a service to the patients and they expect to receive a quick and efficient service. Therefore patients can, in a sense, also be seen to be becoming consumers of the informatics resources as technology connecting them to their healthcare records improves. Good informatics is beginning to develop, patients are beginning in some areas to use imaging data to understand their diagnosis and the rationale for treatment. Therefore, the process of imaging acquisition and sharing must be conducive to patient education within any given clinical setting.

Evolving Producers

Clinicians in many ways regard radiographers and radiologists as producers of imaging data, which they then consume. It is important to understand the evolution of our producers. Radiographers of the past were responsible for image acquisition in accordance with the clinician's request. However, modern teachings encourage radiographers to act as the patient's advocate by filtering and adapting requests to ensure adequate clinical information is provided to warrant the investigation and potential radiation. This is one of the reasons why the UK terminology of a radiological referral is 'request' rather than the USA preferred 'order'. Within the UK there is a common saying: 'You order a pizza, you request an X-ray', which reinforces this. Clinicians must embrace this change in producer autonomy and the new culture that encourages communication between the producers and consumers. Feedback from consumers to producers is still extremely limited in many workplaces: an optimum solution would be as shown in **Fig. 12.3**.

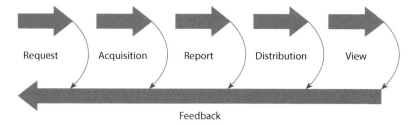

Fig. 12.3 Proposed dynamic relationship between consumers and producers.

Current Frustrations

Government policies and healthcare funding necessitate that hospitals are run effectively as businesses and therefore each hospital chooses its own (or as part of a commissioning group) electronic records, pathology, and imaging systems based on cost versus functionality assessment. The lack of one unifying system between all healthcare institutions is a constant source of frustration for both patients and clinicians. Patients often share their surprise and disbelief that healthcare systems in the UK lack integration, given that information sharing has become a major part of modern society.

Image acquisition has dramatically improved over the last 10 years and this has had a profound impact on the speed and accuracy of the decision-making process, but more importantly has improved patient care. However, the discord between the limited integration of current systems utilised within our healthcare system despite the perceived capabilities of modern digital systems is the main frustration shared by clinicians and patients alike.

Image Sharing

Image sharing still remains an ongoing issue among clinicians. Digital images are easily viewed on computer terminals throughout the hospital; however, the ability to view these images off-site or at another hospital requires electronic portals to transfer the images. The use of these portals adds to the administrative burden of clinical and non-clinical staff and often leads to delays at the bottleneck points in the clerical process of organising the transfer. The temporary storage of these images at the recipient location often leads to situations where patients are being reviewed at the secondary hospital but the original transfer has expired and been discarded. This often leads to local re-imaging being required, which wastes resources, is not strictly compliant with legislation, and leads to dissatisfied patients.

Another area of current concern in the UK clinical community is from those who are not on site during their on-call shifts. These more senior off-site clinicians rely on their juniors (based in the hospital) to convey the appropriate information over the telephone regarding the clinical situation in order to request and obtain imaging, as well as their interpretation of the imaging, possibly for a patient they have never met owing to the practice of shift patterns. Many clinicians feel (incorrectly) there is no universally used system that allows images to be transferred to the consultant at home using existing technologies. Viewing stations at home or remote connectivity would be potential solutions; however, this would require funding and resources that often are the limiting factors in such changes, as well as the guarantee that the data would be adequately protected. To overcome this barrier, Snapchat, iMessage, and other single-use instant message services are typically used to take a photograph of the imaging on hospital workstations, then relay to the external clinician, purely in order to progress patient treatment. This is obviously an unsatisfactory arrangement with large confidentiality and quality issues; however, many hospitals choose to turn a blind eye to the practice owing to lack of other permanent solutions.

Along with viewing off-site, complex cases that require a specialist opinion are referred to tertiary referral centres. With the NHS practice of centralisation of resources to provide specialist treatment, referrals to tertiary referral centres are now frequent and common practice. To enable this, radiological images and history are transferred through the UK's national IEP from the referring hospital to allow these images to be reviewed at a MDT meeting by a group of specialists well versed in managing such complex cases. This system of image transfer is crucial for this referral and review process to work effectively. The disadvantage of the current IEP system is the administrative burden it places on the junior members on the team. The cumulative time devoted to requesting IEP transfers and drafting referral letters is time that could be used elsewhere towards clinical matters. A central repository of images would enable this process to be more fluid and minimise the preparatory time devoted – the technology needs to develop to being more seamless, mobile, immediate, and universal. From a clinician's perspective, their own role is to gather information, make decisions, and treat patients – patient care should not be compromised by simple repetitive administrative tasks, such as those involved in sharing images.

The Ideal Relationship

The perfect synergy between clinical practice and imaging informatics would be the seamless synapse between demand and production, to enable clinicians to freely discuss cases and make complex decisions with minimal administrative burden. The ability to share images instantaneously via a dedicated, secure incarnation of sharing portals, such as WhatsApp or Snapchat, would allow remote senior support over difficult decisions to be provided within seconds. The use of such portals would rely on adequate screen resolution to make accurate clinical plans from the imaging then made available.

MDT meetings are one of the most expensive meetings healthcare institutions can hold – these should be conducted like a virtual boardroom meeting, with the referring clinician present in the decision via remote access. A unifying system that provides access to imaging results and pathology results in one portal would also facilitate this MDT approach. The establishment of such a system will ultimately increase and improve the quality of the time spent with our patients once it has been adequately integrated into services.

Overall, patients entrust us with their health and wellbeing, and therefore we must remain up to date, connected, and share information effortlessly. Our social world is connected like never before, and we should strive for the same degree of integration in our healthcare system. Imaging informatics is a vital part of this and requires well trained and informed staff to operate and maintain those services, plus engagement from suppliers to develop meaningful solutions.

CHAPTER 13

INFORMATICS AND THE WIDER COMMISSIONING ENVIRONMENT

Public Sector Procurement

Public sector procurement covers the purchasing of almost everything the public sector (including state healthcare systems, such as the NHS in particular) requires. Whether it is a full-blown replacement PACS or routine clinical supplies, a process in accordance with specific regulations is required. The relevant regulations (in the UK) are the Public Contract Regulations 2006 or the Public Contracts (Scotland) Regulations 2006, which comply with the European Commission Consolidated Directive on Public Procurement (2014/24/EU). These are intended to ensure all procurements are as fair and transparent as possible and that value for money is obtained.

When we think of 'value for money' (commonly abbreviated to VFM) we often consider buying something at the lowest possible price, but within clinical care there are wider aspects of the clinical service to be considered. While cost is important, the quality and specification of the product, plus the lifetime ('whole life') costs of the purchase must be assessed. If a decision is made to buy goods that are not the cheapest, the decision has to be justifiable and defendable against challenges from other competing suppliers (who may be aggrieved at the loss of sales).

In these circumstances, the added value of the chosen goods or services must be clear and recorded against a set of evaluation criteria.

In order to begin a procurement, the evaluation criteria of any product or service must be pre-defined and issued to the prospective suppliers at the time of tender. This will set out both the financial criteria and the non-financial criteria.

Examples of financial criteria could be:

- Capital cost.
- Maintenance costs.

Examples of non-financial criteria could be:

- Compliance with specified standards.
- Lifespan.
- Ergonomic design.
- Compatibility.

The criteria used and their relative weighting will be down to local preference and should be documented.

The Procurement Directives and the corresponding UK regulations are listed in the *Official Journal of the European Union* (*OJEU*). The *OJEU* is the journal of record for the EU published in a number of official languages of the member states. The *OJEU* is no longer published in hard copy version and it can be accessed online for free via the internet, with suppliers having access to other premium features at various costs. European Directives set out detailed procedures for public sector purchases or contracts whose value equals or exceeds various financial thresholds.

In addition to these regulations, procurement in the NHS is also governed by the individual organisation's standing orders and standing financial instructions (SFIs). These set out the value at which a quotation, multiple quotations, or tender process is required. These are unique to each specific purchaser so can be obtained locally for examination.

Procurement Overview

The taxpayer expects the Government to spend tax revenues wisely and to achieve VFM; this is particularly important in a time of financial austerity. Public sector organisations collectively spend over £150 billion a year on the goods and services they need to fulfil their objectives.

In order to achieve good VFM, public sector procurements need to be efficiently and effectively managed, well planned, and delivered to budget.

Most imaging informatics professionals will at some time be involved in radiology-based informatics procurement. As there are rigid rules that govern how the public sector procures goods and services, the procurement process is comparatively complex and it is always wise to seek experienced support. There are common steps that informatics professionals (themselves managing millions of pounds of software and equipment) should be aware of as a minimum. For healthcare institutions, informatics procurements will often require a significant investment, plus the product or service chosen will need to be proven safe and effective as well as designed in a way that meets local 'human' approval (user friendly). The pressure to deliver the project into radiology successfully will place a significant resource pressure on the procurement team and informatics professional, so pre-emptively gaining an insight into the process will reduce pressure during the intense project phases.

The major IT elements within an imaging department are the PACS, RIS, display monitors and workstations, networking, plus any specialist viewing applications. When planning a procurement, consideration should be given to items such as:

- The technology currently available.
- Technological developments being planned.
- Matching service need with system availability.
- The type of contract required.
- Longer-term service arrangements.
- Migration and archiving plans.
- Workflow patterns/changes expected.
- Level of skill of the PACS team (or those undertaking daily housekeeping/maintaining the service on site).
- Level of experience and authority of the project team.

The list is long and complex, more so if a regional (multi-Trust) procurement is contemplated. The actual process of procurement should not be rushed and should be expected to take far longer than suggested.

Low-value purchases (replacement diagnostic monitor, additional workstation, additional licences, etc.) are typically dealt with internally, based on a single quote (potentially from an existing supplier), with just a management line authorisation escalation on eProcurement systems depending on the standing financial instructions currently in force.

Medium-value purchases are also typically handled internally, requiring several quotes and an internal 'discussion' before authorisation.

High-value purchases are required to be advertised and follow an official procurement pathway. Individual Trust processes should be consulted to find out threshold values (which may change frequently depending on the financial condition of the organisation).

There are currently four official procurement procedures for high-value purchases:

1 The negotiated tender (with a call for competition). This procedure has limited use, primarily when a single supplier is believed to be the sole source of the exact products required (often because of patent protection) and no other similar options for supply are believed to be available. Alternatively it may be used when exacting and precise specifications need to be negotiated, or for cases of extreme urgency. Owing to these, it is not extensively undertaken by imaging informatics professionals, and will not be discussed further.

2 The open procedure. With this a notice is placed in the *OJEU* with a requirements list (essentially a 'shopping list'). All suppliers who respond to the notice indicating interest are instructed to return a tender by a certain date. All tenders are evaluated before the contract is awarded. This procedure does not allow any form of pre-qualification or pre-selection and so is primarily where a specific requirement is needed, and usually the cheapest price is all that is required (e.g. 10 of model xyz monitors, including 20, 2 m HDMI cables delivered by 1st January). However, this procedure can result in an overwhelming number of responses.

3 The restricted procedure. This allows for screening of potential suppliers to ensure those bidding have suitable experience and resources. A notice is placed in the *OJEU* with the requirements list, suppliers responding to the notice are typically asked to complete a questionnaire (a PQQ or pre-qualification questionnaire). From this a short-list is drawn up, with the short-listed suppliers then being invited to respond to an invitation to tender (ITT). The contract is awarded based on the tenders received; there is no opportunity for negotiation. This is a relatively concise two-stage process in which a short-listing system can be used to prevent suppliers without provenance hijacking the procurement by submitting an artificially low bid. This procedure is discussed in more detail later.

4 The competitive dialogue procedure. This is used for more complex procurements, or procurements where the requirements cannot be fully defined at the outset and perhaps local customisations to workflow are required. The selection process between suppliers who respond to the *OJEU* notice involves a two-way dialogue between the parties and ultimately the outcome is agreed between both parties. The final award is based upon this agreed set of outcomes. This is a commonly used procurement method for radiological purchases, and is expanded upon later.

Restricted Procedure and Competitive Dialogue Procedure

As the two most common processes for imaging informatics professionals to be involved in, the next section will give an overview of the restricted and the competitive dialogue procedures. As informatics procurements have the potential to be high risk, with complex solution specifications and significant technical challenges when integrating into an operational clinical department, it is essential that planning is commenced early and reviewed often.

Restricted Procedure

For complex procurements, the Restricted Procedure (**Fig. 13.1**) is usually too inflexible as it incorporates only limited discussion with suppliers. It is used in situations where three conditions are met:

■ The needs of the procurement are well defined.
■ There may be a number of suppliers who believe they are able to meet the buyer's needs.
■ The procurement is not for a grossly customised service or product.

By using this procedure the buyer has the advantage of limiting the number of suppliers invited to tender for the contract by setting minimum criteria relating to technical, economic, and financial capabilities,

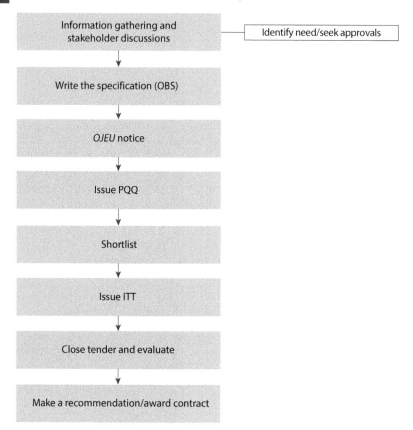

Fig. 13.1 Flowchart of a typical restricted procedure procurement process. (ITT, invitation to tender; OBS, output-based specification; *OJEU, Official Journal of the European Union*; PQQ, pre-qualification questionnaire.)

which potential suppliers must satisfy. Following evaluation and short-listing, a minimum of five suppliers (unless fewer qualify) are invited to offer a tender (present a final price and specifications).

Competitive Dialogue Procedure

The competitive dialogue procedure (**Fig. 13.2**) is more flexible than the restricted procedure and is particularly useful where the

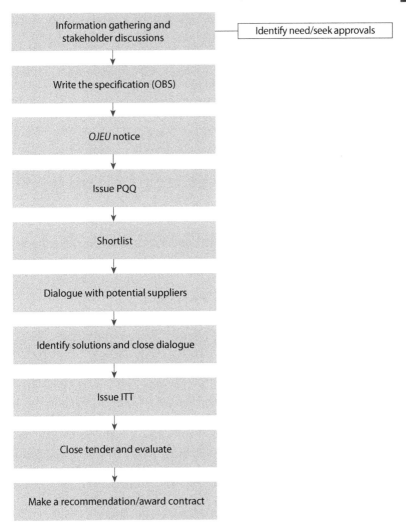

Fig. 13.2 Flowchart of a typical competitive dialogue procedure procurement process. (ITT, invitation to tender; OBS, output-based specification; *OJEU, Official Journal of the European Union*; PQQ, pre-qualification questionnaire.)

contract will have a medium to high level of complexity. It allows dialogue between purchaser and suppliers, which resolves the issue of the buyer at the outset not fully understanding the technology currently available to satisfy its needs and requirements. A similar pre-selection exercise is undertaken as takes place in the restricted procedure, with potential suppliers being short-listed; however, dialogue follows to develop the procurement request further. This dialogue benefits the buyer (who can learn more about what is possible and what should be procured, by having input from a range of suppliers, including their experts and sales personnel) and also the sellers (who can negotiate project requirements, which may advantage themselves against competitors). Once dialogue is complete, suppliers are asked to submit a formal tender based on the updated requirements.

Ultimately, as the stages across both methods are similar, the key portions are detailed here together.

Output-Based Specification

Effective planning is essential for any procurement, and this takes place with stakeholders (staff or users involved or affected by the projects output – the new PACS/the new monitors, etc.). Simplified, an output-based specification (OBS) is a checklist of wants and desires for the purchase. During pre-procurement planning and preparation, the procurement project team (known as the project board) can identify its needs by consulting with stakeholders. The OBS produced is required to contain enough detail to enable suppliers to understand the project's requirements but it should not be so excessively descriptive as to stifle any opportunity for innovation. The balance of the two extremes, plus identification of any constraints and associated risks, should also be given due consideration from the outset. It should be noted that stakeholder engagement may well be an iterative process (as users begin to think about what is required, and what they personally want), with sufficient time and resources being allowed for the completion of a clear and unambiguous OBS. For standard commercial off-the-shelf (COTS) products, 'stock' OBS are available as templates, saving time.

Leading from this, the input of stakeholders is crucial. There are many parties who will be interested in the procurement, often for different reasons. For example:

- The procurement must meet the needs of service users; these are often users outside the Radiology department, e.g. clinicians in A&E, intensive care, clinics, GP practices, or private providers.
- The investment must satisfy the financial constraints of the organisation.
- It must meet the wider organisation's strategic objectives and goals.
- It may need to satisfy those with an interest in integrated working and/or the joining up of data flows across the wider healthcare community, such as neighbouring internal departments (in many cases, pathology imaging can easily be stored on a radiology PACS for example, but rarely can cardiology imaging, owing to the differing types of data structures utilised).

Stakeholders are often identified as part of the business case process, which precedes the procurement process, being led by the project manager in charge.

There are a number of key questions to consider with stakeholders:

- What is needed?
- Why is it needed?
- When is it needed?
- What budget is available?
- What solutions exist in the current open market?
- What will be the key performance indicators?
- How will we migrate to the new system?
- How will it integrate with systems in place within the organisation?

The answers to these stakeholder questions should shape the OBS and define what the project wishes to achieve; consequently it is vital to ensure the necessary multi-disciplinary expertise is available not only to evaluate the procurement process but also to execute the resulting plan.

Window shopping (known as 'pre-market engagement') is often the most effective method to understand the solutions available. It is always important to engage with suppliers prior to beginning the procurement process in order to understand what technical options are currently available, and what is upcoming and being developed.

It should be noted that once a procurement process has formally commenced, all supplier engagement must be managed under the auspices of the process, and no informal supplier contact should be undertaken. In general it is strictly forbidden and a cause for summary (immediate, indefensible) dismissal to accept gifts, tokens of appreciation, or offers from suppliers (including expenses payments, travel allowances, and hotels) unless all suppliers are offered the same opportunity and the amount is reasonable plus an expected part of the procurement process, such as for a local site visit to see software in live clinical use. Radiographers involved in procurements should be extremely aware of these restrictions, as their regulatory body (Health and Care Professions Council: HCPC) may become involved if there is any question of even accidental impropriety during procurements.

PQQ Stage

The PQQ is used to establish the suitability of prospective suppliers to provide the contract in terms of competence, capacity, and capability. It ensures that contracts, and with it public money, are awarded to the most legitimate, capable companies that are robust and financially sound. The detail of the PQQ is at the discretion of the buyer, but it should focus on the technical and/or professional capability, financial and economic strengths, and eligibility of the suppliers. It is important that the assessment criteria and relative weightings are clearly defined in the documentation to avoid later challenge by disgruntled 'losing' suppliers.

In the context of informatics procurement, it may be helpful to use the Trust or Health Board's website for publishing all documents to help prospective suppliers and reduce email traffic, plus for large procurements (of PACS, image archives, display hardware, etc.) it may also be beneficial to hold a suppliers, open event to bring prospective suppliers together on a single day to answer any common queries as one.

Following receipt of the PQQ, the next step is to evaluate the suppliers' responses to identify the qualifying companies. A scoring matrix comprising the evaluation criteria and weightings is completed for each submission. The team evaluating the PQQ must have the necessary skills to assess the supplier responses from a technical, clinical, and business perspective. Financial accounts of each of the potential suppliers should also be assessed in order to determine the economic and financial standing of each interested company, to reduce any chance of insolvency part way through the project. Following this evaluation and 'short-listing', the buyer produces an evaluation report, which identifies the reasons for rejecting suppliers. Each supplier has to be advised in writing of the outcome of the PQQ evaluation stage.

When following the competitive dialogue procedure, at this point the purchaser can enter into a number of rounds of discussions and negotiations with suppliers, with increasing clarity and definitions being made (negotiations are not permissible using the restricted procedure). This leads to the ITT.

ITT

After a short-list has been chosen, the suppliers will be issued with an ITT document, providing an unambiguous statement of requirements including key performance indicators. Evaluation criteria and weightings are also published with enough detail to enable a fair assessment and comparison of the received bids. The suppliers then submit their tenders to a deadline and they are assessed against the criteria. Once this assessment has been done, the chosen tender is recommended to the project board, and feedback must be given to those rejected.

Guidance on the Public Contracts Regulations 2015 and requirements on PQQs are readily available from UK Government websites, plus individual healthcare institutions will each have local policies, which can be consulted. The above EU procurement process has been long standing in the UK; however, following the UK vote in 2016 to disengage from the EU many laws, including those around procurement, may change over the print life of this text. Given the volume of UK laws currently tied to long-standing EU directives, the withdrawal process is likely to take several years, and no changes are currently expected for the foreseeable future. Experience shows though, that it is likely that towards the beginning of the 2020s the public sector procurement process may change to reflect the UK no longer having the same ties with the legislation originally creating the above process. Imaging informatics professionals who are reading after the UK has completed its withdrawal from the EU should check with their institution's procurement department for any changes.

Alternatives to *OJEU* Procurement

OJEU procurements are, as can be seen, complex. As an alternative in specific cases, commonly purchased items can also be purchased via pre-formed framework agreements. Under such an agreement, goods or services are evaluated by a centralised third-party broker and, if they satisfy specific criteria, are added to a framework (in this context, a framework is effectively a list of things for sale). Providers set out their terms and conditions in advance and purchasers can make specific purchases known as 'call-off contracts'. A framework agreement does not commit any party to purchase or supply, and it itself is also governed by legislation. Expert advice must be sought in order to make use of them. Note that there is the potential for framework providers to charge comparatively high percentage 'arrangement' fees that may or may not be transparent to the purchasers. In some cases, the effort of undertaking an *OJEU* procurement can bring higher value results (higher specification, more licences, better functionality, lower ongoing maintenance costs, etc.) for the same cost when comparing with a framework offering.

CHAPTER 14

INFORMATICS AND THE LAW

THERE ARE TWO TRUTHS IN MALPRACTICE CLAIMS

- The MEDICAL truth: what actually happened.
- The LEGAL truth: what the court will decide happened, on the basis of evidence and what has been recorded at the time...

Data + Context = Information

Modern and developing technologies continue to change the risks that healthcare staff need to consider on a daily basis in practice; for radiographers, PACS and RIS have had a large impact – they allow (almost) instant access to hundreds of thousands of records and millions of images. *Data* acquired as part of patient examinations (such as images, or reports) *plus* the *context* in which the data sit produces *information*. It is this information that informatics exploits in various manners.

From 1971 until 2016, the legal owner of all patient data in state healthcare institutions (including medical records and radiographs) was the UK Secretary of State for Health who held copyright and delegated guardianship of patient data to individual Trusts. The effect of devolution led in 2016 to the ownership of patient data being transferred from the UK Secretary of State for Health to the health minister or health board in each of the devolved regions in England, Wales, Scotland, and Northern Ireland, again with guardianship delegated to individual institutions. In practice this means that while they do not 'own' the data, the PACS Manager (or equivalent) is responsible for compliance with the various laws governing the use and safe storage of data handled and generated in the imaging departments by their systems.

Information Governance

Information Governance (IG) is an umbrella of guidelines and principles to help practitioners gather, use, and look after information. It has the following four key areas relating to patient data:

- Making sure it is complete and current.
- Available when required.
- Access safeguarded.
- Using informatics tools with the information to benefit patient care.

The Department of Health considers IG to include the following responsibilities:

- Holding it *securely* and *confidentially*.
- Obtaining it *fairly* and *efficiently*.
- Recording it *accurately* and *reliably*.
- Using it *effectively* and *ethically*.
- Sharing it *appropriately* and *lawfully*.

In order to achieve this, several initiatives are in place. For example, every healthcare practitioner within NHS England is required to carry out annual IG training in a similar manner to Basic Life Support, Health & Safety, Fire & Evacuation. For many years this has been delivered via the online Information Governance Training Environment (IGTE) website. The IGTE training consists of a modular set of training units customisable to the level of involvement with patient data and information each practitioner is exposed to. Modules include:

- Password Management.
- Information Security.
- Secure Transfers of Personal Data.
- Business Continuity.
- Risk Management.
- Caldicott Report Recommendations.

Information Types

In the context of healthcare informatics, there are four types of information we need to be aware of:

1 Confidential.
2 Personal.
3 Sensitive.
4 Anonymous.

1 Confidential information is private data (not publically available) AND given to somebody with a duty of confidence AND expected to be used in confidence (such as a GP consultation). *There are limited exceptions (such as crime/abuse).*

2 Personal information is anything that identifies an individual (e.g. name, address, date of birth, telephone number).

Note that NHS number, H&C number/Social Security/Tax/National Insurance identifiers, or some hospital numbers on their own are initially categorised as data, but can be considered personal information if the correct context is known (as Data + Context = Information applies). Scottish CHI numbers are considered personal information as they contain the individual's date of birth; other hospital numbers may also include dates of birth or other demographics and so are additionally identifiable from the outset. In some cases, even with a name removed, if the rest of the information is 'infamous', such as a widely-reported case in the media, it remains personal.

3 Sensitive information has a stronger legal protection as this type of information can be used to discriminate against an individual. It includes:

- Ethnicity/religious beliefs.
- Political views or opinions.
- Health.
- Sexual/mental health.*
- Criminal records.*

---

* Joint highest potential for harm if unlawfully disclosed.

4 Anonymous. To make information anonymous, it must be unidentifiable and detached from the source and this is achieved at different levels:

- Anonymisation converts the information into a form where it is difficult to identify the source individual; within radiology this is typically done by removing demographic information from DICOM files.
- Pseudonymisation leaves information traceable to source but only by those holding the contextual data – widely used for clinical trials.
- Deidentification is the highest level of detachment; deidentification removes both visible and non-visible clues as to the origin; this may for radiology imaging include selective depth blurring or pixilation of distinctive anatomical features, such as the face on CT head studies – preventing high-resolution CT scans from 'giving away' otherwise anonymised data sets.

It is important to remember that automated anonymisation tools, including those used during CD/media export routines bundled with many common PACS providers, may only by default anonymise technical parameters they recognise and have been programmed with in advance. In many cases additional technical parameters (particularly private DICOM tags) are included with image sets that are non-standard and so are not removed in many cases. This has led to accidental identification in some cases – exported anonymised images must be manually verified using an application capable of exposing the underlying stored details in the image's DICOM headers to be sure that no identifiable data remain. Anonymisation is an unsuitable technique if recipients of the data have prior knowledge of details of the original data (perhaps as a research study candidate), as it would be simple for the removed details to be restored by the third party in these cases.

Caldicott Principles

Patients in the UK expect privacy and discretion. In 1997, owing to the increasing use of IT to manage patient records, a report was commissioned (known as the Caldicott report after its author Dame Fiona Caldicott), with revisions in 2012 (Caldicott 2) and 2016 (Data Guardian Review). A senior staff member within each healthcare institution must be nominated as a Caldicott Guardian, with responsibilities including organisational compliance with the recommendations and best practice. The key responsibilities for all staff handling patient data are:

- To justify the purpose(s) for using patient data.
- Not to use patient-identifiable information unless it is absolutely necessary.
- To use the minimum necessary patient-identifiable information.
- To access patient-identifiable information on a strict need to know basis.
- That everyone should be aware of their responsibilities to maintain confidentiality.
- To understand and comply with the law, in particular the DPA and GDPR.

Regulations

The primary legislature handled within a Radiology department on a daily basis has long been IRR99 and IR(ME)R 2000. At the time of going to print, both regulations are being reviewed, with the replacement IR(ME)R anticipated to come into force in the first few months of 2018. Likewise, updates to IRR99 are also being consulted upon, with an expectation of a revision released shortly afterwards.

In the context of informatics, the proposed updates have the effect of strengthening the requirements on stringent data recording within the imaging speciality.

Additional legislation should be considered beyond these when managing an imaging informatics service. Further key regulations that must now also be considered by the imaging informatics professional include:

- Freedom of Information Act, 2000 (FoIA);
- Data Protection Act, 1998 (DPA) or from Spring 2018, its replacement: the General Data Protection Regulation – EU Regulation 2016/679 (GDPR);
- Access to Health Records Act, 1990 (not commonly abbreviated);
- Bribery Act, 2010 (not commonly abbreviated).
  (Note: due to Scottish law varying from English & Welsh law, there are similar but differently named legislations affecting Scotland.)

The FoIA (2000) applies to all public bodies (NHS Trusts, schools, councils, governmental bodies, etc.) intended to force 'openness', preventing unnecessary secrecy and allowing stored information to also benefit patients. The intention of the regulation was to inspire trust and confidence that data collected from patients were 'doing good'. The FoIA provides that everybody has a right of access to information held by public bodies – any person can request statistics or data held by a public body that is not covered by the DPA (i.e. personal data is not requestable using the FoIA, as this would actually be covered by the DPA instead).

Until its replacement in 2018 by the GDPR, the DPA 1998 forms a large part of IG, enshrining in law certain basic requirements, with the Information Commissioner's Office (ICO) overseeing compliance in the UK. The Act requires the implementation of appropriate technical (and organisational) measures to protect personal data against accidental, unauthorised, or unlawful processing, destruction, loss, damage, alteration, disclosure, or access. Everyone who is responsible for using data is required to follow strict rules called *data protection principles* as outlined in the DPA. Summarised, these are that the information is:

- used fairly and lawfully;
- used for limited, specifically stated purposes;
- used in a way that is adequate, relevant, and not excessive;
- accurate;
- kept for no longer than is absolutely necessary;
- handled according to people's data protection rights;
- kept safe and secure;
- not transferred outside the EU without adequate protection.

The DPA covers not only patient data, but also corporate data and staff data. All breaches of the DPA are reportable to the ICO who investigates, with fines for breaches being common (but more of concern is the inevitable public 'shaming' and predictable newspaper articles that accompany this).

The new EU-wide GPR, is in broad terms an extension and expansion of the DPA, taking into account the new uses of personal data on the internet and the processing possibilities of ever more powerful computer systems and algorithms. The GDPR has the aim of requiring data handlers to build in high levels of protection by design and default, with data portability requirements and formal nomination of

Data Protection Officers being incorporated in the new regulations. In addition, new rights are also created for individuals and new specific responsibilities for data processors and controllers plus new types of personal data are defined that were not foreseen at the creation of the older DPA some 20 years prior (for example, an individual's biometric or genetic profiles).

The new personal rights created for data subjects (the people who the data is about) by the GDPR are:

- The right to be informed.
- The right of access.
- The right to rectification.
- The right to erasure.
- The right to restrict processing.
- The right to data portability.
- The right to object.
- Other rights in relation to automated decision making and profiling.

To address rising concerns over misuse of personal data aggregated from multiple sources over time or the unauthorised disclosure of data (loss through hacking being an example), levels of additional accountability, governance, and breach reporting requirements are also introduced. Significantly heavier financial penalties for breaches, plus an inherent requirement for all processing activities to be continually secured to prevent malicious or unintentional data leakage round up the bulk of the changes between the DPA and the GDPR.

Radiological data sharing is one regularly utilised area in which legal considerations are paramount – while all clinicians and the clerical staff based at other institutions will be pressuring for the most rapid transfer method possible, it is critical that in any such transfers, whether electronic or physical, adequate safeguards are taken. Along with the duties surrounding keeping patient data confidential, it is good practice to ensure that all radiological data transfers are necessary, justified, and proportionate, together with records being kept allowing audit of each individual transfer. These records could be maintained on the RIS or OCS for accessibility and should include as a minimum, specific details of:

- What data were sent.
- When.

- To whom.
- Who requested the transfer.
- Why they requested the transfer (the reason and justification for the transfer).

Two other areas of concern surround online cloud storage, plus separately offline data backups for disaster recovery – both of these services are utilised in different manners, but both require consideration against the principles of the original DPA and GDPR, in particular the need for safe and secure storage within the EU.

The Access to Health Records Act 1990 has almost entirely been repealed. Its remaining provisions dictate the process for access to deceased relatives' records, including radiological images and reports.

The IR(ME)R 2000 regulations (and newer revision) exist to ensure that any radiation received by a patient will potentially be of benefit to the health of the patient and will be optimised. It is therefore important that informatics systems allow for healthcare practitioners to determine and record:

- The examinations have undergone a justification procedure (perhaps also vetting or checking protocols if required). This is particularly influenced in modern practice by the availability of rapid image transfer services presenting a need to check if a similar examination has occurred at another institution, to which an image transfer request can be made rather than re-irradiating the patient unnecessarily.
- Dose records (or detailed exposure factors) – monitoring and optimisation of patient doses is an ongoing process and by comparing individual results with local and national 'diagnostic reference levels' (DRLs), techniques utilised in the acquisition of images can be adapted accordingly.
- A clinical evaluation of the outcome of each exposure in accordance with the employer's procedures. This is most commonly a report.

IRR99 (and also its newer revision) influences informatics to a lesser extent, but still requires its support for equipment quality control and maintenance requirements.

When handling procurements or suppliers more generally, those involved with imaging informatics should be aware of the requirements of the Bribery Act statute. Some systems, particularly VNAs at present, are high-profit margin items, and suppliers may be tempted to offer incentives for those with purchasing influence (including PACS team members) to gain exposure to their commercial offerings. The Bribery Act 2010 formalises the crime of giving or receiving bribes in a commercial context. 'Bribes' are defined in the widest sense, with meals, travel expenses, or items that would otherwise be considered trivial included – it is always a necessity for those in the PACS teams to consult local 'gifts and hospitality' policies and make regular declarations as suppliers make their approaches (even if in informal ways) to avoid later challenges.

Social Media

Prevalent in modern society, the use of instant messaging and social media presents great challenges in complying with legislation surrounding confidentially. Younger patients are ever keener to share their every movement, including when receiving healthcare treatment. With the advent of miniaturisation, radiographers and practitioners are reminded to be aware of patients undertaking filming or covert recording on handheld devices. This is especially important, as it is exceptionally difficult to clear a working area within a Radiology department of confidential material (whether it be a stack of request forms for scanning, a list of portable X-ray examinations outstanding, theatre schedules on a whiteboard, modality worklists, or simply open tabs detailing prior patients on the PACS viewer or PC). For this reason, it is strongly recommended that photography by patients or their relatives is not permitted in clinical areas. It is important to introduce this point to students who, mainly being part of a generation used to sharing social updates, may not foresee the dangers of allowing this behaviour, and therefore are at higher risk of being exposed to patients asking for a quick 'selfie' or photograph of their radiographs by mobile telephone camera for souvenir purposes far more than previous generations of radiographers were. During the life of this text, the Social Work and AHP regulation body (HCPC) is intending to publish social media guidelines for all registrants.

Figure 14.1 shows a reproduction of a genuine Facebook posting (by a patient), inadvertently exposing four prior patient details (listed on the 'open window' tabs of the PACS image viewer) plus details of 16 patients on a handwritten radiographer's paper theatre scheduling list (beside the console keyboard).

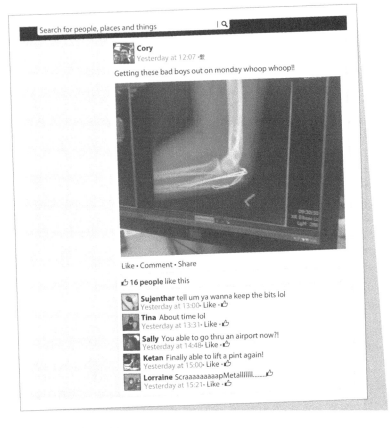

Fig. 14.1 Breaches of data protection owing to radiographers allowing patients to take photographs in the clinical workspace.

Informatics Policies and Procedures

SOPs are a library of regularly updated system policies and procedures to ensure that staff have a current unambiguous point of reference to follow when undertaking either routine or non-routine tasks. They are traditionally the responsibility of the PACS Manager or their deputy to maintain.

Sample SOPs for an acute NHS institution may include:

- Standard guides on common usage pathways for each system.
- Pathway for users to report system faults.

- Pathway for users to report abnormal clinical events, such as cancer referrals/A&E unexpected findings.
- Permissions and parameters for the acceptance of electronic requests from external (non-radiology) systems/referrers.
- Business continuity and DR guides detailing 'fall-back' workflow in the event of particular failures.
- Details of clinical governance arrangements.
- Routine housekeeping lists and responsibilities.
- Rest scripts.
- Removable media import/export policy.
- Document scanning and retention policies.
- User access control (including who is entitled to request user accounts and what training is required).
- The process for identifying students, agency, and temporary staff from permanent staff.
- Audit and statistics report lists.
- Process for systems training and validation prior to escalation of privileges.
- Data sharing arrangements.
- Standard responses to commonly asked patient queries.
- Data or task dictionary (to ensure standardisation).

Human Factors

Humans are frequently found to be the 'weak link' in any process involving IT.

The two main aspects relating to informatics in this discipline are safety and system integrity.

Safety

Many PACS manufacturers certify and regulate their systems to national standards as for medical devices in the EU, and consequently, just as with syringe pumps or anaesthetic equipment, PACS should only be operated by competent and trained people.

General informatics software supporting informatics in the NHS also are required to comply with Information Standards Board (ISB) notices ISB 0129 (relevant to suppliers: *Clinical Risk Management: its Application in the*

Manufacture of Health IT Systems) and ISB 0160 (relevant to informatics professionals and Radiology departments: *Clinical Risk Management: its Application in the Deployment and Use of Health IT Systems*).

In short, the burdens on informatics professionals are to ensure the correct training regimens are in place and easily accessible by users (which will include those outside of the Radiology department, such as clinicians, other AHPs, students, agency staff, and community workers), plus that software is properly assessed and deemed 'safe' and compatible. Both of these responsibilities are local to the workplace concerned and are difficult in practice to outsource or shift onto a supplier.

System integrity. Many of the regulations require records to be kept complete and current. Achieving this can be as simple as training staff in the relevant systems use and providing them access, but also, just as important, is how to protect records from damaging changes, be that through incompetence or malicious intent.

Forced log-off times. Humans are by nature curious beings, and there is a great tendency now for any unattended hospital PC to be at risk of unauthorised access by members of the public or staff. In the majority of cases, this use is as innocuous as collecting their own emails, the weather, reviewing train times (or at the extremis checking in for a flight). However, some individuals pride themselves on making an example out of those who practise lax security principles, with the media unfortunately supporting them in making examples out of those institutions found insecure. Those organisations handling celebrities or other 'VIPs' (politicians, sports personalities, or even relatively unknown corporate personnel) may also find themselves at risk of monetary enticements to find out specific facts on that person's care. Under the DPA, Systems Managers themselves have the over-riding duty to ensure confidential patient data remains secure, and so this is the reason almost all IT systems, including PACS and RIS, should enforce a user log-off after a period of inactivity (*Table 14.1*). For radiology, guidance was given by Connecting for Health during the onset of the NPfIT programme (summarised below). In practice, clinicians will always pressure for open-ended access, including for radiology systems. To this extent exceeding a maximum recommended time is possible, but ultimately responsibility for the consequences falls onto the System Manager making the change – justification on the necessity of exceeding the maximum

Table 14.1 Recommended and exceptional inactivity log-off times for radiology clinical applications

Area	Examples	Recommended inactivity time before log-off	Exceptional maximum inactivity time before log-off
General public access: no physical security/barrier between the workstation and the public	Ward PCs, reception desks, tablets, handheld devices, portable workstations (workstations on wheels)	5 or 10 minutes	15 minutes
Controlled public access: door (may not be locked, or may have simple push-button code) between workstation and public area	Clinic consulting rooms, ward offices, clerical offices	15 minutes	30 minutes
Secured access: access-controlled door between the workstation and the public area	MDT rooms, consultants' offices	30 minutes	40 minutes
Restricted access: two access-controlled doors between the workstation and the public area	Sterile zones: theatres, isotope preparation	2 hours	4 hours

MDT, multidisciplinary team; PC, personal computer.

should be documented and discussed with the local Caldicott Guardian to establish if the workflow requiring the exception is acceptable or whether safer methods to achieve the same goal are possible.

Student and agency staff. Given that these groups of staff are typically working either under supervision, or have less experience with the systems than substantive staff, consideration should be given to indicating their status in RIS or PACS. In some areas this is achieved neatly by assigning a prefix to their login or identifier code, e.g. AGExx for agency, or Sxx for student, providing a quick visual clarification of the status of the staff member at the time of the examination, even after several years have passed.

Access and user accounts. Access to IT systems is another area where there is typically conflict between clinical staff and Systems Managers. For PACS, owing to the wealth of confidential information stored, it is generally accepted that only staff with the need to directly view the images for diagnosis or progression of treatment should be granted access to the system (e.g. radiology staff, general clinicians, nurse practitioners, plus other AHPs, such as physiotherapists and speech and language therapists). This mitigates against non-practitioners from using their logins to allow multiple other staff access throughout the day (e.g. it was previously common for a ward clerk or general ward nurse to log onto PACS on a ward PC solely for the purpose of allowing multiple clinicians to access throughout the day – defeating audit trails and other access controls completely). Allowing such unfettered access is now considered lax practice on the part of Systems Managers and non-compliant with the DPA principles.

There are multiple international standards to help guide the control of access to health information, including ISO 22600:2014 (Health informatics: Privilege Control and Roll Based Access); but common sense approaches, as below, provide simple starter points.

- Change default passwords on CR readers, portable X-ray devices and block access for generic sign-on accounts (e.g. how many GE-brand DDR mobiles across the country still have the factory default unlock code as 1-2-3-4?).
- Ensure good quality encryption is utilised for remote viewing of PACS images (security along these lines was only introduced into the DICOM standard in 2000).
- Develop and provide quick and easy access to secure image sharing or collaboration tools for clinicians (or they will use inappropriate tools, such as Snapchat or Whatsapp).
- Do not allow users to accumulate higher permissions than is required for the execution of their duties – those with System Administrator privileges (particularly the power to delete images or edit system logs) should be trained and placed under contract with disciplinary weight available for misuse.

- System Administrators should maintain a second 'standard' account for use when they are not performing administration duties, such as when working as a standard radiographer.
- Train users about phishing, viruses, and social engineering techniques.
- Ensure SOPs are up to date and used by staff.
- Robustly organise access control to clinical systems (e.g. careful consideration should be given to certain groups of staff members requesting access to PACS – are they requiring access to view and diagnose patients themselves, or simply to provide a 'generic' login for other clinical staff, thus disrupting audit trails? This can be most clearly seen at the ward level, where non-practitioner nursing or clerical staff rarely have need to access PACS themselves, but are frequently asked by clinicians to share access.).
- Strongly enforce disciplinary consequences for any breaches in policy related to account misuse.
- Provide regular training opportunities.
- Audit system logs for irregularities often.
- Ensure users are fully aware that 'anonymising' rarely truly deidentifies radiological images from PACS.
- Be aware of social engineering techniques and the possibilities of targeted cyber-attacks on radiology informatics systems and infrastructure.

Owing to the increasing number of cyber-attacks on NHS infrastructure in recent years, from a UK-wide perspective, CareCERT (Care Computer Emergency Response Team) has been available from Autumn 2015 (provided by NHS Digital), offering to help improve cybersecurity defences in healthcare institutions by providing proactive advice and guidance about the latest threats and security best practices.

BASIC PRACTICAL TIPS THAT CAN BE ISSUED TO NEW STARTERS OR STUDENTS

Do

- Choose strong passwords and change these in line with current local policy.
- Check you are speaking to the right person when talking about a patient (porters/wards/nurses).
- Be sure you have patient consent before talking to relatives.
- Be careful when exporting images, or talking about memorable cases (location/privacy) – every image has 'hidden' ID headers!
- De-identify/anonymise data properly – be careful of pseudonymisation or incomplete anonymisation.

Do not

- Share passwords.
- Put confidential waste (request forms/reports) in 'normal' waste.
- Leave forms/paperwork laying around.

Best practice for radiographers

- Use an approved encrypted USB stick when transferring data.
- Do not take photos in a hospital (who or what is in the background?).
- Remember email generally is not secure (NHS.net to NHS.net is, plus some others).
- When using images for presentations include the minimum identifying information possible.
- Report incidents promptly (quicker = easier investigation).
- Know where your local policies/procedures are.
- Do not let patients take photos of images.
- Students have the same responsibilities as qualified staff.
- Never be afraid to ask for advice.

CHAPTER 15

THE IT DEPARTMENT'S PERSPECTIVE: PROVIDING A SAFE AND EFFICIENT IT SERVICE 24/7

Enterprise Integration and Service Management

When delivering any IT service, including those used to support radiology, there are additional requirements beyond the boundaries of the system in question itself. For example, reporting staff may be convinced they prefer one particular brand of application over another due to look-and-feel, but there is a far deeper level of consideration to be undertaken in order for these systems to remain operational and useful. This 'background' work is mainly carried out by the staff who are commonly found in the institution's basement (the IT department). For example, even for a simple office productivity suite (the most common in the NHS being Microsoft Office), a key consideration is whether this should be installed locally on each workstation, or perhaps a cloud-based version should be utilised instead. Expanding on this example – if installing locally, that software suite requires more than just the software to be installed – the application needs to be configured for its environment: at its simplest level, is it a 32bit or 64bit operating system? Is there sufficient memory and disk space? The application must understand the architecture in order to exploit it, such as memory constraints and the number and type of cores available in the processor. For both the locally installed and cloud version, questions need to be answered, such as: how many users can it support or what recovery options are available in the event that the spreadsheet application suddenly disappears mid-way through a complex dosimetry calculation (or perhaps rolls back the annual leave spreadsheet)?

In many ways this simple analogy applies when making decisions about clinical software services, such as PACS and RIS, within the Radiology department as well. There are key principles that need to be considered, such as capacity, performance, availability, and security of the service. Working from the ground upwards, infrastructure is the foundation on which all IT services are hosted; should the application be run locally on the hospital network, hosted on-site in the Trust server room and be managed by the Radiology department, or the IT team? Or, instead could it be chosen to be run from a private, public, or hybrid cloud service? In practice though, this decision may change with the exact requirements of the service, and in many cases local policy or strong feeling from stakeholders or 'key players' may in fact dictate the direction of travel, such as a 'cloud first' policy. Each of the major considerations from an IT department's perspective are to be considered here in turn.

Architecture (where does it run from?)

Local IT departments will typically offer a number of choices to host applications, ranging from dedicated server hardware and storage (commonly referred to as 'pizza boxes') to shared virtualised servers with dynamic storage and memory offerings, such as VMware ESX and Microsoft Hyper-V offerings (commonly referred to as 'blades', albeit slightly misleadingly). Well-configured virtual infrastructures are more compact in physical size, and have been found to be more than capable of running most applications as optimally as the dedicated physical alternative. They have also been found to also offer far more cost-effective options for 'high availability' (remaining available even when some duplicated components begin to fail) plus allowing for the provision of common services, such as load balancing. Load balancing is routinely used for high-traffic applications, such as PACS, and is simply where data are shared across multiple components, avoiding saturation, sharing load plus providing fault tolerance and failover capabilities if needed. Failover capabilities help maintain a 24/7 service, automatically switching to a 'copy' system in the event that a whole server or single component fails, preventing unscheduled downtime. High availability often also extends failover capabilities to include scalable or 'elastic' services that can automatically adapt to changing demands, such as increased processor workloads or an increase in the numbers of users, without adversely affecting the availability or performance of the service.

Many of these high availability and scalable options are readily available via cloud service providers (CSPs) even with the most basic of offerings, and have in themselves made CSPs a first stop for large scale public-facing web services. Cloud services usually fall into one of the following categories:

- Software as a service (SaaS).
- Platform as a service (PaaS).
- Infrastructure as a service (IaaS).

The National Institute of Standards and Technology provides helpful definitions for each of these, and in essence each determines how much of a service the cloud provider takes on (and where the responsibility of the local IT department ends). For example, the common Microsoft Office 365 application is a SaaS service – as a customer you have little interest in the infrastructure or platform that sits behind it, you simply pay a subscription and expect the service to be available to you as required over the internet. PaaS is a service designed to allow rapid coding and deploying of applications without any concern for the infrastructure they sit on as this is already provided by the cloud vendor – examples include Google's App Engine platform (which allows you to build scalable web applications and also a mobile backend). IaaS, in comparison, is more akin to traditional IT services in that the buyer has access to the entire infrastructure, such as servers, storage, networks, and operating systems, but these are owned and maintained by the cloud provider. IaaS allows flexibility to create a bespoke environment to exacting specifications while paying for only what is used (as opposed to paying for everything if this was built and hosted on site, as was traditional).

In a clinical setting where large complex data are in use, such as high-resolution images (often referred to as unstructured data) thought should be given to the end-to-end architecture. As is true in most cases, performance will be determined by the weakest link in the infrastructure chain, such as network 'bottlenecks' or single cross-site links. IT departments will sometimes forget or be disinterested in analysing performance of radiology applications (owing to the clinical/non-clinical domain cross-over), but this is in actual fact an important part of optimising radiological applications in live use.

Licensing

Licensing is a consideration that traditionally slips the attention of Radiology departments when purchasing applications – if any application is a third-party COTS product, such as a 3D-reconstruction application or a statistics database, then considerations will need to take place around licensing, in particular if the application requires additional licensing in some environments.

Common types of software licensing include:

- Per number of server processors.
- Per x slices (CT slices processed simultaneously).
- Per modality.
- Volume (amount of use).
- Site size (number of examinations processed per year).
- CALs (client access licences – concurrent users).
- Standalone (requires a 'pizza box' server of fixed determined size/power).
- Enterprise level (for the entire institution, but may not include home/remote access).

Certain types of application, such as business warehouse/statistical analysis software, require one type of licence for creating reports (read/write licence) and another for running the reports to obtain processed data (read-only licence).

In the UK, common RIS vendors typically license their products on a per-volume basis (x number can be logged on at once; or x installs can take place) based on the sizing of the department in question. Common PACS vendors have a greater range of licensing options, many choosing to provide different tiers of licences on a per concurrent workstation basis, e.g. a low level 'basic' licence, a medium-level licence with MPR/3D included, and a high-end licence for specialist features, such as breast imaging, advanced MRI processing, and PET fusion display.

Security

Local IT departments will apply their own security policies and most will, as a minimum, meet the ISO27001 Information Security standards, among others. They will be responsible for ensuring the security of all data held within their local network ecosystem. Any solution procured and deployed by the Radiology department will need to meet these established principles and likely integrate with existing access control systems, such as Microsoft Active Directory (the 'Windows Login'), to manage user access.

CSPs will also offer assurance and service level agreements (SLAs) in relation to the security of their infrastructure and core services.

Common generic threats to an IT service are listed in *Table 15.1*.

While human issues are generally the most common, including those that severely disrupted surgical procedures in a major northern UK teaching hospital in 2016, cyber threats, such as the top three items in *Table 15.1*, are a very real and important point of security management in the NHS. Many people will have been familiar with news stories reporting 'hacks' that liberate personal data from various embarrassing websites; or the impact on patient care that came from the major outbreak of the Conficker virus in many large Trusts across the country in 2008, and even more recently from the very widespread WannaCrypt ransomware in 2017. As Radiology departments are in the habit of importing CDs, USB sticks, and other removable media items in order to bring outside radiological imaging onto our systems, staff and systems need to be well prepared and secured against attacks. Medical staff, under time pressures, are more likely to miss warning signs of an attack in progress or override anti-virus alert messages if they obstruct their use of underlying clinical applications. Understanding that cyber threats are becoming more directed and more complex requires hospitals to stay ahead of the hacker's game – many organisations are

Table 15.1 Major risks against an IT service in the Radiology department

Risk	Primary attack vector(s)	Potential key effects	Mitigation
Malicious software application (commonly: virus/ransomware)	Primarily social engineering (at present)	Leak of confidential data, delays to service, loss of access to data	Policies, training, security software, network monitoring
Intrusion	Hacking	Leak of confidential data, delays to service, loss of access to data	Network hardening, monitoring, penetration testing, and review
Vishing/phishing	Social engineering	Leak of confidential data	Training
Sabotage	Internal, disgruntled employee	Delays to service, loss of data	Policies, permission reviews
Human error	Lack of professional competence	Leak of confidential data, delays to service, loss of data	Training, error disclosure (incident reporting and review)
Breakdown	Hardware/software/infrastructure failure	Loss of or delays to service, loss of data	Redundancy, backups
Reputational damage	Incorrect use of social media, malicious whistle-blowing	Loss of funding	Training, transparency of actions, policies

opting for combinations of security information and event management (SIEM) solutions and intrusion detection systems (IDS) that can provide near real-time monitoring techniques to identify known patterns and apply a level of intelligence to reduce false-positives in virus and intrusion identification.

The choices made in developing the architecture to support the application will vary depending on the volume of users, location, internal corporate policy, and of course budget, but these must be a consideration on top of the main concern of 'which PACS do the radiologists like the best?!'.

Standard Support Framework

A good number of imaging informatics professionals may believe the burden of service management exists solely with the supplier whom they have contracted to provide second-line and third-line technical support (known as a 'managed service'). This sadly ignores the day-to-day realities and environment in which the software is to be running, where the need for effective first-line support will become apparent, and presents a fallacy should external assistance always be relied upon.

Traditional levels of helpdesk support are known as:

- *Self help:* from frequently asked question (FAQ) lists, wikis, help files, etc.

- *First-line support:* provide the initial contact to the end-users and are trained to handle the most common queries received, followed by knowing the correct escalation contacts for more complex or technical matters.

- *Second-line support:* handle escalated queries requiring more time or knowledge to resolve, escalating to third line if the issue appears to be new or novel.

- *Third-line support:* handle the most complex queries as well as previously unknown errors. These personnel interact heavily with developers and research teams to better the software/service in the long term.

For a common PACS team within the UK, first-line support to end-users is typically provided by the keen and knowledgeable radiographers in each department; the PACS team then provide second-line support and finally suppliers are called upon to deliver third-line support. Suppliers themselves will have their own first-, second, and third-line support teams, depending on size of the organisation. Key omissions in some Radiology departments are the consideration of 24/7 support for imaging informatics applications (even though general IT departments are working towards providing 24/7 cover across the board) and too rapid escalation to third-line support (suppliers), which removes the potential for local learning opportunities, together with elongating the resolution process if the problem is quickly shifted externally.

IT Service Management

As we live in a rapidly changing world, delivering new systems is a key part of work in an IT department. The benefit of an IT system, however, is unlikely to be realised until after it has been used for some time and so it matters how an IT system will be supported as it begins to be used more representatively. For these and other reasons the IT departments prefer not to consider solely IT systems, but IT services (or even business services – as IT systems do ultimately now enable businesses to carry out their functions).

In terms of supporting an IT service, including those specific to imaging, there are important considerations.

- Is it clear how users obtain assistance should they have difficulty using the software?
- Is it clear how basic tasks (setting an account up, etc.) can be accomplished quickly?
- If the software ceases to operate, how serious a problem is that – who needs to know and what sort of response is required to put it right in a timely manner?

The most common service management methodology utilised in the UK is the Information Technology Infrastructure Library known as 'ITIL®' (ITIL®v3), which is well established with more than a million people having studied it around the world. ITIL® itself is process based – taking a simple specific case, a user trying to use an IT service has had something go wrong; what do they do? How does the support team respond to this? The methodology recommends a service desk to act as the single point of contact, and a process called *incident management*, which structures the response plus enables the issue to be sorted out efficiently. Within imaging, the service desk will most likely be the PACS office. ITIL® also provides processes for action when the same task repeatedly fails (*problem management*); and after the cause of the problem with a solution is identified, the *change management* process provides guidance on how to implement change safely. Many other processes exist within ITIL® in order to provide standardised functions in managing suppliers, technical operations, capacity, lifecycles, availability, or services in general.

Tight regulatory controls surrounding a safety critical or life-support system cause problems for organisations that wish to innovate at the cutting edge of technology. For one such organisation, continuity of service is critical with the processes and behaviours supporting this. For another organisation, speed plus capability to try things that may fail are priorities, resulting in different approaches. However, the common core of service management is to have a service desk, an incident management tool, a CAB plus first-, second-, and third-line support teams.

The emergence of cloud-based services also prompted organisations in the late 2010s to review how they manage their IT services (as an example, owing to its monolithic nature, Google Cloud services will never use a hospital's change management process even if they host a PACS in the future, but will rather use their own processes, which may differ). The management of multiple suppliers and general increase in system complexity also continues to stretch people's understanding of how to organise services – service integration and management (SIAM) is one approach being explored by future-scoping IT departments to bring those areas more in control.

As IT service management has continued to evolve at differing rates depending on the uptake of new technologies, experiences can be shared by professionals in this area by utilising one of the international chapters (branches) of the IT Service Management Forum (ITSMF). These chapters exist to define standard roles, provide guidance on baseline skillsets for staff (e.g. with the Skills for the Information Age index), and provide routes for interprofessional development. These interactions are particularly important as the move from IT departments doing 'everything' to relinquishing control to cloud or off-site providers or even imaging departments takes place over time.

Project Management

In a similar vein to how ITIL®v3 is utilised as a standardised approach to service management, Projects in controlled environments version 2 (PRINCE2®) is the standardised project management methodology developed and approved by the UK government, and widely utilised within the NHS (and elsewhere) when projects are required. Within the domain of imaging informatics, PACS Managers and other professionals in charge of clinical systems, such as PACS, RIS, and EPR, will find it most useful to have some grounding in the basics of PRINCE2® in order to communicate effectively (in the same 'language') plus understand the stages and processes that are followed as part of the progression of a project. PRINCE2® is a process driven management methodology comprising of 7 principles, 7 themes and 7 processes.

The *7 principles* are:

1 Is the project justified (i.e. does it make sense from a 'business' perspective)?
2 Learn from experience (lessons learned are invaluable).
3 Define roles and responsibilities (detail who should be doing what).
4 Manage the project by stages (such that there is not too great a burden at one time, and that progress can be monitored in measureable steps).
5 Manage by exception (calculate tolerances and place limits on people's authority – allow the project to run within these, but follow-up with checks if stages run outside).
6 Focus on products (the output and delivery – primarily quality and quantity).
7 Tailored to suit the environment (small, simple projects, such as a PACS office refurbishment with few staff affected, has less risk and requires less complexity; a large, complex project, such as a full PACS replacement with multiple external stakeholders in different departments as well as both technical and clinical faces with large risks, requires more planning and control).

The **7 themes**, utilising the 7 principles are:

1 Business case (justification and authority to proceed).
2 Organisation (how is the project/project team organised – who has power to make decisions and is responsible for them?).
3 Quality (assessing whether outputs are fit for purpose).
4 Planning.
5 Risk (identify and eliminate or manage the inevitable risks).
6 Change (many plans require changes part-way through – how are these to be raised and handled?).
7 Progress (how this is monitored, fed back, and graded?).

The **7 processes** are the 'timeline' of the project, in order (which use the principles and themes to populate them):

1 Starting up a project.
2 Initiating a project.
3 Directing a project.
4 Controlling a stage.
5 Managing product delivery.
6 Managing stage boundaries.
7 Closing a project.

The PRINCE2® methodology includes prompts for the creation of many standard documents, such as risk registers, project briefs, lessons learned, and issues logs, which become most helpful as the project progresses. Depending on the size of the project, such documents may simply be single tabs on a spreadsheet application, or may be more formal structured documents for larger endeavours.

As it is so extensive, many imaging informatics professionals choose to study PRINCE2® at Foundation or Practitioner level, with a multitude of training providers existing to facilitate this.

Programme Management

PRINCE2® provides standardised guidance on the progression of projects; however, in an enterprise environment, multiple projects may be running at once, e.g. the replacement of a CT scanner and its connections, a PACS application software upgrade, plus a refresh of virtual reality (VR) hardware. Each of these multiple projects runs independently, but has interactions and, crucially, dependencies with each other. These dependencies may be technical (interfaces and the like), or physical (human resourcing or access issues). This is much the same as in domestic life, where individuals have their own day-to-day 'projects', but a 'programme' is required to oversee as and when those projects are required to interact and influence each other. For example, looking for a larger house would be a project, searching for a higher remunerated job would be another, and the two would need to be managed as a programme if purchasing the house was dependent on a higher salary, and accepting a new job depended on location! Programme management is therefore the process of managing several related projects, often with the intention of improving an organisation's performance. In practice and in its aims, it is often closely related to systems engineering, industrial engineering, change management, and business transformation. The standard framework for managing programmes in the UK is the Managing Successful Programmes (MSP®) framework.

Risk Management

Risks are present in every activity we undertake in life, and are particularly important to recognise when related to clinical software such as that used by radiographers and radiologists. An international standard, ISO 31000, defines risks as 'the effect of uncertainty on objectives'. Within the responsibilities of imaging informatics professionals falls the task of identifying, quantifying, and mitigating (or removing) risks related to the processes they manage. This is particularly important for PACS, as the majority of PACS are operating (and certified) as medical devices; however, the healthcare environment is becoming an ever more complex and litigious place. Management of Risk (abbreviated 'M_o_R®') is the UK's standard best practice guidance for risk management and provides more detail on strategies that should be followed by those in this area.

CHAPTER 16

EDUCATION USING A PACS

While the primary day-to-day usage of a PACS is to store and display imaging for clinical care, the systems do have uses in educational contexts. Healthcare staff are required to be trained as students, then continue training as they gain experience and progress their career as part of continuing professional development (CPD). Modern advances in technology allow many more options than have been previously available in the era of film and chemicals.

Historic Educational Methods

The impact of technology on education has been seen in teaching and learning from pre-school to university – it is perhaps only 30 years ago when blackboards and OHPs were omnipresent in the classroom. Medical and radiography education has benefited considerably from the technology and it is imperative that the technological advances within the world of clinical practice are replicated within the education setting to ensure students are prepared for the demands of their chosen profession.

The history of informatics in education represents a fascinating journey that moves from large, cumbersome computers and calculators via the PC and laptop to the smart phones and tablet devices of today. There have also been moves within the education sector to diversify from the traditional lecture presentation to be more intuitive. Each one of these advances provides an interface between the student and learning their chosen profession in a style that is more spontaneous and bespoke for the individual learner. While advances in technology have assisted many students in learning, when introducing new learning technologies universities and education providers need to be aware of their legal responsibilities in terms of equal access and students with specific educational needs.

Virtual Learning

Many of the changes in education instigated by technological advances can be applied across many areas of education and are not specific to medical imaging. Of particular significance is the advance of the virtual learning environment (VLE). In previous generations, lectures and tutorials would have represented the only opportunities for learning, and any absences would have resulted in the experience being lost. VLEs permit students to learn remotely via the internet without the time restriction that a lecture timetable would give, giving rise to the concept of 'distance learning'. Rather than simply a repository for lecture presentations, VLEs can also be used as an assessment tool, to track engagement and encourage communication and collaboration in learning. VLEs tend to operate under a licensing arrangement between the educational institution and learning system provider, either purchased directly, are open source (such as the Google provided 'Moodle' platform), or even developed within an institution for their own bespoke needs.

In addition to, and sometimes embedded within, the VLE is the ePortfolio. Previously, professional development would have been documented within a paper file; however, advances in technology mean that experiences can be documented, reflected upon, and shared digitally as with many other documents. Within the UK, the Society of Radiographers developed its own ePortfolio (named 'CPD Now') to assist its members in their CPD accreditation. Given that CPD is regarded as mandatory by the UK regulatory body for radiographers (the HCPC), recording of experiences is vital in maintaining competence and ePortfolios can be regarded as a more up-to-date method of documentation.

Practice Simulation

The notion of simulating clinical practice within the education setting is not a new one. The desire to give students a safe experience to practice their clinical skills without fear of harming a patient is entirely understandable, but the experience must be sufficiently realistic for the learning experience to be beneficial.

Technology advancement has allowed the creation of realistic simulated patients that can accurately replicate a clinical situation and whose apparent physiology can be controlled remotely by teachers. While not specific to the clinical application of radiographic technique, simulated patients give opportunities for radiographers to learn about medical emergencies and the deteriorating patient. Post-radiological contrast media anaphylactic shock is a situation that could arise in the career of a radiographer and provides an example of the experience that simulated patients can replicate. Radiography educational institutions typically house their simulators within a realistic clinical skills suite that is designed to replicate a real clinical experience; augmented reality is a recent development, facilitating the use of 3D image recognition via a tablet device to display videos depicting real life patients related to the simulated patient's physiology. In addition to adult simulation (**Fig. 16.1**), child and neonatal simulators also exist to replicate experiences in the paediatric setting.

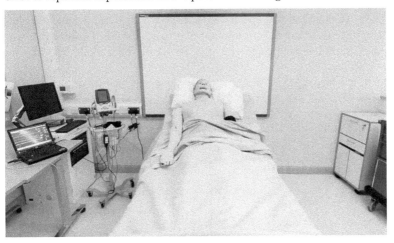

Fig. 16.1 A simulation model patient 'Sim Man'.

The simulation of radiographic technique is complex and there will be many that argue that there is no substitute for the reality of imaging of real life patients. However, VR can provide additional practice opportunities for students away from the pressure of a busy clinical department.

One of the earliest examples of VR in the setting of medical imaging in the UK came with the advent of 'VERT', a VR training system in radiation therapy. VERT provides a 3D depiction of a Linac treatment facility that seeks to improve student's psychomotive skills in the treating of patients. The DICOM-compatible format makes it possible to import bespoke treatment packages providing a link to genuine clinical practice.

Within diagnostic imaging, 2007 saw the advent of a virtual radiography simulation for diagnostic radiography, mammography, and fluoroscopy (by a company called Shaderware – **Fig. 16.2**). The system is a combination of three distinct computer simulations together to create a realistic platform for the diagnostic radiography student who wishes to develop their clinical imaging techniques. The software seeks to join classroom and clinical learning by creating an interface that can be used by teachers within a classroom setting as a demonstration of good practice, or by the student in their own time.

Similar technology exists in relation to the use of fluoroscopic equipment (C-arm) in the operating theatre, which is traditionally a challenging environment for radiographers to operate in. Training packages that intended to bridge the gap between theoretical training and

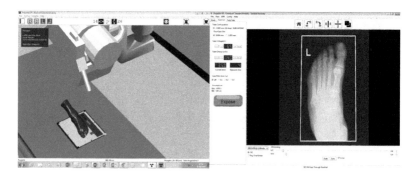

Fig. 16.2 Overview screen of virtual radiography simulation software.

practical application of C-arm operation do exist but do not appear to be in widespread use in the UK at present.

One of the greatest benefits of utilising VR in the setting of medical imaging education is that the simulation is performed without subjecting patients to unnecessary doses of radiation. The intention is that accurate replication of clinical imaging and therapy can reduce technical errors within clinical practice that can lead to repeat imaging.

In a wider clinical and more interprofessional setting, virtual communities now exist that blend realistic depictions of service users within a varied community setting. By creating a virtual community, education providers can create patients with complex medical needs, which can link different strands of medicine, including imaging and rehabilitation. This allows the student to appreciate the patient journey more rather than the specifics of imaging alone.

Anatomy Teaching

Cadaveric dissection accompanied by artistic depictions in text books were the mainstay of anatomy teaching for centuries. The advent of radiology changed diagnostics but also the way anatomy could be displayed. This has further evolved into more computer generated, 3D, and cross-sectional imaging, and it is vitally important that anatomy in an education setting mirrors the experience that occurs within clinical practice. Challenges have arisen over the modern ethical use of cadavers and this was the catalyst in developing alternative technologies.

While traditional methods of anatomy teaching should not be consigned to history, new technology permits new ways to educate and allows students different platforms to improve their learning of this vital subject. The advent of computers and CDs allowed students to have their own learning resource they could access without attendance at lectures or dissections. This has now further developed via tablet devices to anatomy applications, which are available for download, or web-based resources that allow the student not just to view the anatomy but interact with it as well. Touch-screen technology and increasing computer memory now allows students to display the anatomy in ever increasing detail and manipulate the anatomy in more ways.

Even though the teaching of clinical anatomy is relevant across different disciplines, displaying of radiological anatomy represents more of a niche market for imaging professionals. With the limited market and the amount of data that are required in imaging, most of the generically available anatomy applications do not routinely include radiology, despite the blending of clinical and radiological anatomy being important for both medical students and those training in medical imaging. Several of the practice simulation software packages have elements of anatomy within them, but packages that are purely designed to teach anatomy are a more recent phenomenon and have owed much to improvements in display equipment, so that interactive anatomy can now be displayed more clearly and in a larger, more student friendly format.

Anatomy visualisation tables (**Fig. 16.3**) operate in a similar manner to a tablet device with a touchscreen interface but on a much larger scale. Utilising a common clinically connected table, users can access clinical anatomy atlases alongside a library of 'real' (but de-identified) patient cases, along with live patient imaging if desired. Primarily utilised for clinical MDT meetings, from an educational context these tables can be used both for teaching anatomy and pathology and are considered a much more versatile option than was available with

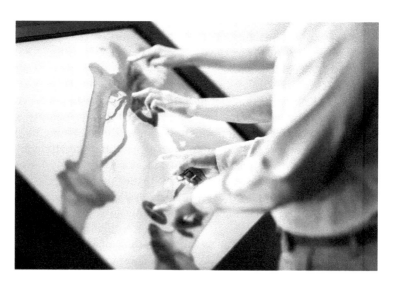

Fig. 16.3 MDT meeting and touchscreen education table.

previous technology. The use of wireless network connections allows new cases to be shared on a global scale, with students also being able to obtain remote access to cases via an education portal on the internet. For anatomy tables, radiologically the focus is on cross-sectional imaging and 3D rendering of the body parts, but images from other imaging modalities, histology, and photography can be imported for comparison and case enhancement purposes. The tables are also designed to complement clinical dissections when appropriate, replacing the traditional visits to the mortuary that were a common feature of the undergraduate curriculum until recently. A further benefit of anatomy visualisation tables is that they can be used to assist radiography students in understanding how anatomy is affected by patient positioning. As with others aspects of informatics within education, the widespread adoption of standards, such as DICOM, has been vital in the ability to transfer images for teaching purposes between different locations.

Image Interpretation and Reporting

A shift in attitudes to image interpretation being undertaken by non-radiologists has been observed in clinical practice over recent decades, with radiographers being the frontrunners in this shift of attitudes in terms of career progression and opportunities for role expansion. For these processes to occur effectively, changes were needed at both undergraduate and postgraduate academic levels to reflect increased image interpretation requirements. At a time of film-based imaging, educational institutions needed to develop a library of images to support its students; in the age of digital imaging, an electronic archive of cases is needed to facilitate teaching plus an array of devices to display them on (**Fig. 16.4**). As image interpretation for radiographers has moved from conventional radiography to other imaging modalities, the archive needs to reflect the type of image interpretation being provided by the institution. One of the biggest challenges faced by universities is therefore creating their own archive. Some may have links with local imaging departments who may permit access to their PACS; however, legislation on data protection and the rigorous application of it can make access to real patient images stored within a hospital PACS challenging. The need for de-identification is paramount and it can be

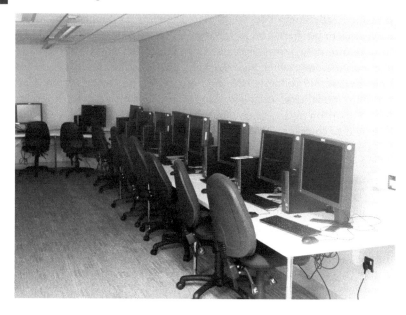

Fig. 16.4 A university-based, educational PACS suite.

felt that even the presence of significantly unique pathology can be sufficient to identify a patient.

Universities require PACS similar to those found within the hospital environment, with similar compatibility if images are to be uploaded from outside sources. In addition, image viewing conditions need to be broadly similar to those within clinical practice. This would include both background in terms of uniform viewing conditions, quality of workstations, and other factors normally unique to the clinical environment.

To reflect increased radiographer involvement in cross-sectional image interpretation, it is important that educational institutions have the software that can display images in different formats. Free image processing software, such as OsiriX, has been developed for the navigation and viewing of multi-dimensional images. The increased use of multi-planar format and volume rendering in clinical imaging means that the universities who seek to provide training in cross-sectional image interpretation would benefit from being able to depict such images within their own institution. Such imaging facilities could be used in conjunction with other faculties outside of health, such as archaeology or forensic science, to provide an educational resource that can benefit students other than just those that study radiography or medicine.

Informatics has impacted dramatically on imaging services and it is vital that education keeps pace with this impact to ensure the professionals of the future are sufficiently equipped for the demand. It is also important for teachers to appreciate the different learning styles and learning needs of their students, and be able to adapt teaching to meet those needs. Having a range of resources can help in terms of diversifying teaching, but should come with a warning. Equity of access and teaching in a non-discriminatory manner should not be overlooked, particularly when using new technology that pre-emptively assumes certain levels of competence in IT.

There is no substitute for actual clinical experience in terms of developing many skills, but the ever advancing evolution in informatics has permitted teachers to diversify their teaching in areas such as technique, anatomy, and image interpretation beyond the traditional and into a very modern world. It is therefore important that teachers continue to be aware of technological advances within the field of imaging informatics and education to maintain their concordance with current best practice.

CHAPTER 17

PROFESSIONALISM: DEVELOPMENT AND CAREER PROGRESSION IN INFORMATICS

Within radiology, although a misnomer, 'PACS management' has become the accepted generalised term for a particular branch of health informatics, focussing primarily on the implementation and maintenance of radiology and cardiology information systems, typically including the PACS and RIS at its heart.

Radiographers moving into this speciality characteristically also take on additional responsibilities stemming from being the 'IT person' close at hand, a role that also may include troubleshooting workstations, fixing PC problems, changing broken dictation handsets, and even replacing toner cartridges. Traditionally known as PACS radiographers (or, if senior, PACS Managers), their role encompasses many skills similar to that demanded by other specialities in radiology – management of people, resources, technology, budgets, providing training, writing policies, and planning, plus any clinical component that might remain. An alternative background for entry into the profession is via holding experience in IT, having an IT degree and then showing an interest in imaging informatics. The IT method of entry produces a slightly different variety of job titles, such as PACS Administrator, Radiology Systems Analyst, or System Consultant, but with similar roles. This split entry and progression structure also holds true for other departments, such as Cardiology or, more recently, Pathology. Outside of the main acute hospital environment, local solutions, such as for veterinary practices or dentists, frequently also require at least one individual in the practice to take the lead on installing, commissioning, and maintaining smaller scale informatics equipment; with these more contained projects it is important to keep up to date with wider best practice in order to avoid placing the systems (and therefore patients) in jeopardy as practice evolves.

What Do PACS Radiographers Do?

By far the most common imaging informatics practitioners in the UK at present are radiographers who have been given responsibilities in the informatics arena. PACS radiographers themselves can come in many different flavours depending on their experience and formal structure within radiology – generally some will be IT literate radiographers who have gradually built up a reputation for being a problem solver within a department and functioning akin to an application specialist: fixing studies when wrong names are entered, troubleshooting modality worklist failures, and training new staff in the use of CR, DDR, and other software applications.

Other PACS radiographers will have been employed into a senior radiographer role with a specific responsibility for, and time allocated to, PACS, and will frequently carry out the training of new clinicians and the installation of PACS or RIS software, as well as investigating hardware failures and potentially even carrying out the equipment QA.

Stepping up through the ranks, radiographers who become Deputy PACS/Systems Managers take on additional responsibilities, primarily relating to business functions – the formation of departmental system policies, liaising with clinical equipment suppliers to set up new connections or features, and monitoring the system's resources.

At the more involved level, superintendent radiographers working as Systems Managers are typically the leaders of the Radiology department's informatics strategy – these are the individuals who formulate long-term goals, are consulted before new equipment purchases, and who guide the organisation's priorities relating to clinical IT. They hold budgets and financial responsibility specific to the informatics service. The post of Systems Manager is a team leader who uses the support of their staff to effectively run the services and has overall responsibility for maintaining the various systems integrity and availability.

The Five Facets of PACS Management

Breaking down the tasks and responsibilities, five distinct facets can be seen almost universally within the role.

1 IT (technical skills). Covering the three main areas (software, hardware, network) this embraces general matters, such as maintaining team webpages, FAQ lists, managing connectivity issues, fault finding, installation of workstations, and administration of user accounts, as well as ancillary clerical matters, such as stocking printers and ordering supplies. This is in addition to servicing the critical requirements of medical information system equipment: ensuring uptime, speed, availability, integrity, and providing for 24/7 working, as well as provisioning for business continuity and disaster management.

2 Clinical. Manipulation or administration of medical images requires knowledge of the clinical speciality concerned. Housekeeping tasks, such as study administration, merging, matching, unpicking mix-ups, and identifying human errors, are core duties utilising clinical experience. Providing guidance to other modality leads on the purchase of new equipment, such as digital mobile radiography machines, is also critical.

3 Legal and compliance. Compliance with information standards notices, data set change notices, authoring policies, audits, SOPs, managing governance issues surrounding security, user administration, research projects, records retention, subject access, and FoIA requests are just part of this facet.

4 Public relations. PACS teams are a noticeable part of the Radiology department providing a comprehensive service; should PACS be unavailable, the entire department's work is made significantly more challenging. Maintaining IT and vendor relationships plus 'selling the system', managing expectations, gathering feedback, testing, providing information, and in some cases apologising for failures, fall under this facet.

5 Analytical. This facet covers producing and returning mandatory and ad-hoc statistics for national healthcare board purposes, internal audits and registrar logbooks, project management, support for departmental research and development projects, and managing finances (providing advice on large investments: PACS replacements are valued in the tens of millions of pounds in larger sites or regions). Effective project management (PRINCE2®), service management (ITIL®), and people or team management form part of this facet.

Career Progression

There are two distinct direct entry points into the upper 'managerial' sections of the PACS profession: as a qualified HCPC registered radiographer with a degree or diploma working upwards from a senior radiographer, or as an IT practitioner (with or without any qualification) becoming involved within radiology. From either of these starting points, experience of PACS and development of the extended skills necessary allows progression within the field and the related increases in responsibility. After entering the profession there is a general career progression structure from around Band 5 (PACS Radiographer*) to Band 8b (Radiology Systems Manager*), but with no clearly defined, or nationally standardised gradings in between (mostly owing to the varying sizes and needs of each institution).

As with other areas, the themes of skill development for PACS radiographers can be grouped. A generalised career progression flowchart can be created giving the following broad patterns of development (**Fig. 17.1**).

What Opportunities are There?
Formal Systems Training

This is the basic level of training required to be an effective autonomous PACS professional and is unique to the specific applications installed

---
* Titles are genericised.

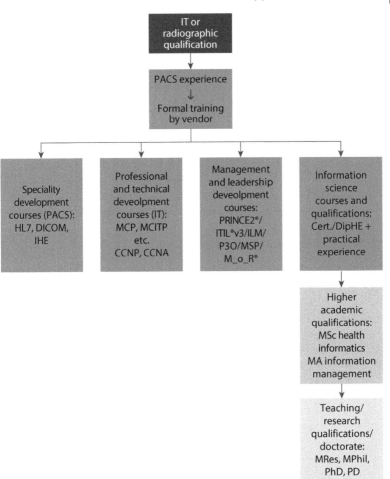

Fig. 17.1 A typical learning pathway for imaging informatics radiographers in the UK. (CCNA, Cisco certified network associate; CCNP, Cisco certified network professional; DICOM, digital imaging and communications in medicine; HL7, health level 7; IHE, integrating the healthcare enterprise; ILM, Institute of Leadership and Management; ITIL®, Information Technology Infrastructure Library; MCITP, Microsoft certified IT professional; MCP, Microsoft certified professional; M_o_R®, Management of Risk; MSP, Managing Successful Programmes; P3O, Portfolio, Programme, and Project Offices; PACS, picture archiving and communication system; PRINCE2®, Projects in Controlled Environments version 2.)

and that need to be managed. This type of training is available directly from the system vendor (Sectra, Insignia, Carestream, Agfa, FujiFilm, GE, Siemens, Philips, etc.), or from outsourced speciality training providers in local clusters. Cascade training can also be offered locally for junior members of staff to disseminate knowledge more rapidly. Collaborative working with other sites also has benefits, e.g. within clinical radiography the topic of cardiac CT has recently inspired many co-operative learning efforts between sites, with some offering more formally organised paid-for courses and others choosing to informally provide a mentoring service to neighbouring sites. PACS radiographers can also take the opportunity to see different implementations of the same or different systems, and to see how workflow differs when additional changes are made (perhaps, for example, when eRequesting for radiological services is rolled out to GPs, or when bronchoscopy/endoscopy/ECG machines are connected to PACS).

Speciality Development (PACS)

Speciality development includes training in the 'basics of the trade', e.g. HL7, DICOM, and IHE. Many new PACS radiographers have just a basic understanding of the standards that underpin the systems used in radiology (and the wider healthcare environment), but even when searching for more information can struggle to find out more owing to the lack of textbooks and easily absorbable guides. Radiology HL7 and DICOM training is available in the UK, which focuses on how the core radiology (RIS/PACS) and other hospital systems (eRequesting, EPR, MPI) 'talk' to each other, and how problems can crop up in the flow of data around the systems. This is a particularly good strand to explore and revisit for CPD as, being related to medical IT, these topics are developing and evolving relatively rapidly as the healthcare community is continually refining them. Keeping on top of these changes is important not only for those radiographers obliged to undertake mandatory CPD, but also for non-radiographic PACS staff who may have to interact with other PACS Managers with different skill levels.

Professional & Technical (IT)

Being responsible for health information systems brings with it the assumed concerns for the supporting equipment. Basic network training (common courses, such as the Cisco CCNP, CCNA, CompTIA or similar), IT support customer service training (any of the many applicable Microsoft certifications), and a grounding in specialist areas such as server virtualisation (training similar to the VMware VCP or VCA courses appropriate to the specific system in use) help greatly with fault finding and the early identification of any potential problems.

Management and Leadership

A large chunk of PACS management duties is related to strategy and forward planning. Having knowledge of sound project and IT service management methodologies (from nationwide short courses, such as PRINCE2®, ITIL®v3, MSP®, and P3O) helps prevent the misuse of scarce resources and ensures the service is running in a documented and auditable manner. Management of Risk (M_o_R®) teaches risk identification and control, highly useful for when product upgrades are offered and their impact is required to be considered in the live environment.

Information Sciences

Much of the informatics profession integrates more widely with other parts of the clinical IT environment within health institutions, and as such has active academic communities across the country. PACS radiographers can develop their information science skills through reflective learning, or by undertaking medium-length diploma level certifications in subjects, such as Informatics or Information Management (readily available across the country).

Higher Academic Qualifications

Leading on from the diploma and certificate level courses, various Masters level qualifications are available that provide a deeper insight into the profession. Many MSc courses include a dissertation allowing the individual to develop their critical thinking and research skills in a topic chosen by themselves. These higher qualifications build on the knowledge of information sciences introduced earlier, to aid in the better comprehension of future requirements and enhancements to the current workflows.

Teaching/Research/Doctorate

Comparatively few radiographers have qualifications above Masters level when compared to other professional groups, such as nursing and physiotherapy. The National Institute for Health Research funding data show that as of 2013 (the latest full data sets available) just five successful applications were declared as being from radiographers from a total of 717 health professionals who completed, or are completing, a nationally funded, in-service, level 8 (PhD) academic qualification, with none of these being clearly definitively PACS related. Alternatively, a Professional Doctorate (PD) in radiography is suitable for those who wish to incorporate more of their clinical work and experiences into the qualification, and receive initial training in research matters rather than immediately dedicate themselves to purely academic study. At doctoral level, education becomes predominantly self-guided and begins to create new knowledge for the profession as a whole, benefiting not only the hosting Trust but others in similar situations. Teaching can take many forms, and is differentiated from standard training or inductions (internal to the place of occupation) by sharing knowledge more widely within the community, for example, by guest lecturing, preparing submissions to peer review journals, or presenting at speciality conferences.

Forming a Functional Imaging Informatics (PACS) Team

Experience across the UK has shown that imaging informatics applications demand a number of dedicated positions in order to correctly maintain the services that they provide across an entire enterprise. As budgets are squeezed, Radiology departments may look to pare positions or freeze vacancies, and given a choice between a Band 6 CT radiographer or a Band 6 PACS radiographer, sadly the choice is not always favourable to the informatics profession. This in many cases leads to a reduction in informatics support with delays becoming evident in the acquisition and reporting process, plus innovative patient care via the delivery of modern technology not being implemented. Imaging informatics is effectively just another speciality within radiology, and should be afforded the same basis for staffing to maintain its effectiveness.

Resourcing and Skill Sets of the (PACS) Team

Offered as an informational guide, as local approaches vary owing to historic practices, *Tables 17.1–17.3* are presented following the analysis of team structures and job descriptions from across the UK in the past decade. Note that in some institutions posts may be split between the Imaging and IT departments, with a consequent reduction in headcount within the clinical environment. Band 8c vacancies additionally do exist, but are extremely rare, with only one direct PACS management post being advertised across the 2 years of authoring this text.

Table 17.1 Large institution (e.g. a multi-site acute Trust with several trauma departments)

Grade (NHS band)	Indicative or representative job title (formal NHS employers' terminology/*Historic pre-agenda for change* (2004) terminology)	Typical number employed (full time equivalent)
3	Image Transfer Clerk (Clinical Support Worker for Image Sharing/*Film Library Clerk*)	1–4
4	PACS Assistant (Assistant Practitioner (PACS)/*PACS Helper*)	1–2
5	PACS Radiographer/PACS Administrator (Radiographer/*Radiographer*)	1–2
6	PACS Radiographer/PACS Administrator (Radiographer Specialist (PACS)/*Senior Radiographer (PACS)*)	1–2
7	Deputy PACS Manager (Radiographer Team Manager (PACS)/*Superintendent IV Radiographer*)	1–2
8a	PACS Manager (Radiographer Principal for Informatics/*Superintendent II Radiographer*)	0–1
8b	Radiology Systems Manager (Radiographer Consultant (PACS)/*Superintendent I Radiographer*)	0–1
Total number of full time equivalent staff		5–10

NHS, National Health Service (UK); PACS, picture archiving and communication system.

Table 17.2 Medium institution (e.g. a single-site Trust or multi-site Trust with a single A&E department)

Grade (NHS Band)	Indicative or representative job title (formal NHS employers' terminology/*Historic pre-agenda for change* (2004) terminology)	Typical number employed (full time equivalent)
3	Image Transfer Clerk (Clinical Support Worker for Image Sharing/*Film Library Clerk*)	0.5–1
4	PACS Assistant (Assistant Practitioner (PACS)/*PACS Helper*)	0.5–1
5	PACS Radiographer/PACS Administrator (Radiographer/*Radiographer*)	0–1
6	PACS Radiographer/PACS Administrator (Radiographer Specialist (PACS)/*Senior Radiographer (PACS)*)	1–2
7	Deputy PACS Manager (Radiographer Team Manager (PACS)/*Superintendent IV Radiographer*)	0.5–2
8a	PACS Manager (Radiographer Principal for Informatics/*Superintendent II Radiographer*)	0.5–1
Total number of full time equivalent staff		3–7

Table 17.3 Small institution (e.g. a low through-put NHS site or private practice)

Grade (NHS Band)	Indicative or representative job title (formal NHS employers' terminology/*Historic pre-agenda for change* (2004) terminology)	Typical number employed (full time equivalent)
4	PACS Assistant (Assistant Practitioner (PACS)/*PACS Helper*)	0–1
5	PACS Radiographer/PACS Administrator (Radiographer/*Radiographer*)	0–1
6	PACS Radiographer/PACS Administrator (Radiographer Specialist (PACS)/*Senior Radiographer (PACS)*)	1–2
Total number of full time equivalent staff		1–4

As recruitment and staffing of imaging informatics teams should be considered in the same manner to any other speciality within radiology, it is important to balance levels of skill, education, and experience appropriately. Imaging informatics is a complex discipline and therefore requires suitably developed staff with an emphasis on the clinical components of the role, along with sufficient IT support. As disruption to a PACS or RIS has wider impacts outside of radiology, larger acute centres should ensure 24/7 internal support is available from the PACS team by provision of a funded on-call rota.

Outside Radiology

In the UK, the main area where rapid growth is currently being experienced is in pathology, a service whose departments are beginning to receive significant investment across the UK to begin the modernisation from manual slide-based processing towards digital pathology. As a result of this, the field of digital pathology is developing in much the same manner as was observed within radiology during the 2004–2006 era of the NPf IT, and in similar ways as imaging departments transitioned successfully away from the analogue film and chemical era. Career pathways for pathology informatics personnel are less formatively defined at present, but appear to be following the same pathway as discussed here.

While Cardiology PACS Managers are fewer in number than Radiology PACS Managers (and indeed some share the role), the skills required are broadly similar.

Organisations of Interest

The entry requirements into the senior levels of the PACS management profession demand high levels of competence in four quadrants: *speciality*, *technical*, and *management* skills (which relate directly to functions with radiology) together with *informatics* expertise (which interfaces the profession with the wider clinical environments). CPD is readily available; however, the onus is on the individual PACS professional to locate and embark on the correct development pathway for their current circumstances and learning preferences. As competition for employment is greater, it is becoming comparatively rarer to obtain a senior position without having undertaken at least some further academic studies.

There are many national organisations that promise to grade, certify, and register information skills either for free or on payment of a fee, but almost none are found tailored for the specific demands and rigours of the imaging informatician. Rather, the individual Informatics Specialist Interest Groups of the respective radiological professional bodies (SCoR, BIR, BCS, and RCR) are good starting points for contact if guidance is required or should individuals have an interest in contributing to the development of the profession. Although Radiology is one of front-running departments in diagnostics for informatics and thus leading the way in many respects, the BCS (being the national institute for IT) has many active groups of other healthcare professionals holding a wealth of knowledge who are keen to share best practice in other areas that are not traditional strengths of clinically-trained staff, such as data security and business continuity matters.

There is an active community of PACS Managers in the UK, and many of the professionals already in posts are usually more than happy to receive requests for advice and interest from those seeking to enter the profession. Remembering that informatics is effectively just another modality in a well-functioning Radiology department should help dispel some of the mystery from around the profession. Indeed, specialising in imaging informatics is roughly the same process as specialising in any of the more 'traditional' (CT, MR, US, NM, etc.) modalities – show an interest and someone will be sure to show you the ropes, grateful for the extra pair of hands! Hopefully this text will have gone some way to reinforcing this.

ORGANISATIONS OF INTEREST

Society for Imaging Informatics in Medicine
(www.siim.org)
This international society covers multiple countries and is headquartered in the USA; it organises an annual meeting and regular international events.

Society and College of Radiographers IM+T Advisory Group
(www.sor.org)
A UK-based group that promotes informatics to the NHS and the private radiography workforce.

British Institute of Radiology Clinical Intelligence & Informatics Special Interest Group
(www.bir.org.uk)
A UK-based, cross-discipline group that brings together radiographers, physicists, radiologists, and registrars.

European Society of Medical Imaging Informatics
(http://www.eusomii.altervista.org/)
An institutional member of the European Society of Radiology that operates in multiple countries.

National Non-Profit Informatics Training Sessions for Radiographers
(www.learnpacs.com)
This often runs training at various levels for staff working, or students interested in, imaging informatics.

Royal College of Radiologists Imaging Informatics Group Forum
(www.pacsgroup.org)
A lively UK discussion forum habited by radiologists and suppliers.

A number of regional PACS mailing lists or groups are also available across the UK; the majority are via invitation from existing members or the requisite group leader (to those engaged in qualifying informatics positions).

RESOURCES

Chapter 1

Department of Health (2002) *Making Information Count: A Human Resources Strategy for Health Informatics Professionals*: http://archive. forumpa.it/forumpa2003/sanita/cdrom/cnr/documenti/making_ information_count_final.pdf (accessed 8/5/17)

Chapter 3

Brainerd EL, Baier DB, Gatesy SM, *et al.* (2010) X-ray reconstruction of moving morphology (XROMM): precision, accuracy and applications in comparative biomechanics research. *Journal of Experimental Zoology Part A: Ecological Genetics and Physiology* **313**(5):262–279.

National Electrical Manufacturers Association (2011) *Digital Imaging and Communications in Medicine (DICOM) Standard Part 3: Information Object Definitions.*

Pansiot J, Boyer E (2016) 3D imaging from video and planar radiography. In: *MICCAI 2016–19th International Conference on Medical Image Computing and Computer Assisted Intervention* (Volume 9902).

Chapter 4

Bauman RA, Gell G, Dwyer SJ III (1996) Large picture archiving and communication systems of the world – Part 1. *Journal of Digital Imaging* 9:99–103.

Bauman RA, Gell G, Dwyer SJ III (1996) Large picture archiving and communication systems of the world – Part 2. *Journal of Digital Imaging* 9:172–177.

Department of Health (2009) *Records Management: NHS Code of Practice Part 2*, 2nd edn.

Chapter 5

Health Information and Quality Authority Ireland (Feb 2010) *International Review of Unique Health Identifiers for Individuals.*

Individual Health Identifier, 2016 eHealth Ireland: http://www.ehealthireland. ie/Strategic-Programmes/IHI/
(http://www.digitalhealth.net/news/47985/individual-patient-identifier-live-in-ireland)

Ludvigsson JF, Otterblad-Olausson P, Pettersson BU, Ekbom A (2009) The Swedish personal identity number: possibilities and pitfalls in healthcare and medical research. *European Journal of Epidemiology* **24**(11):659–667.
http://www.ncbi.nlm.nih.gov/pmc/articles/PMC2773709/

Medicare Healthcare Identifiers Service: https://www.humanservices. gov.au/customer/services/medicare/healthcare-identifiers-service, Department of Human Services, Australian Government

NHS Choices 28/08/2016 *Your Health Care and Records:* http://www.nhs. uk/NHSEngland/thenhs/records/nhs-number/Pages/what-is-the-nhs-number.aspx

NHS Digital, *The NHS Number, Staff Questions*: http://systems.digital. nhs.uk/nhsnumber/staff/faqs

Chapter 6

Chang P (2008) Re-engineering radiology in an electronic world: the radiologist as value innovator. *Applied Radiology:* http://appliedradiology. com/articles/re-engineering-radiology-in-an-electronic-world-the-radiologist-as-value-innovator (accessed 03/02/16)

Colon in CT: A Survey. *IEICE Trans Inf Syst* **E96-D**(4):772–783.

Elevitch F (2005) *SNOMED CT: Electronic Health Records Enhance Radiology Patient Safety*: http://www.auntminnie.com/index.aspx?se c=ser&sub=def&pag=dis&ItemID=66036 (accessed 24/12/15)

Esquivel A, Sitting DF, Murphy DR, Singh H (2012) Improving the effectiveness of electronic health record-based referral processes. *BMC Medical Informatics and Decision Making* **12**:107.

Haug PJ, Pryor TA, Frederick PR (1992) Integrating radiology and hospital information systems: the advantage of shared data. In *Proceedings of the Annual Symposium on Computer Application in Medical Care* (p. 187). American Medical Informatics Association.

Health and Social Care Information Centre (2015) *SNOMED CT:* http:// systems.hscic.gov.uk/data/uktc/snomed (accessed 21/12/15)

HL7 UK (2016) *HL7 Delivers Healthcare Interoperability Standards:* http:// www.hl7.org.uk/index.asp (accessed 19/01/2016)

Itagaki MW, Ripley B, Kelil T (2015) 3D printing and 3D modeling with free and open-source software (hands on) RCB24. Radiological Society of North America, 2015.

Kierkegaard P (2015) Interoperability after deployment: persistent challenges and regional strategies in Denmark. *International Journal for Quality in Health Care* **27**(2):147–153.

Kings Fund (2016) *The Digital Revolution: Eight Technologies That Will Change Health and Care:* http://www.kingsfund.org.uk/publications/articles/eight-technologies-will-change-health-and-care (accessed 17/1/16)

Marr B (2015) *How Big Data is Changing Healthcare:* http://www.forbes.com/sites/bernardmarr/2015/04/21/how-big-data-is-changing-healthcare/#4339276932d9 (accessed 22/01/16)

Murray J, Saxena S, Modi N, Majeed A, Aylin P, Bottle, A (2013) Quality of routine hospital birth records and the feasibility of their use for creating birth cohorts. *Journal of Public Health* **35**(2):298–307.

NHS England/ HSCIC (2015) *Interoperability Handbook.* NHS England, Leeds: https://www.england.nhs.uk/digitaltechnology/wp-content/uploads/sites/31/2015/09/interoperabilty-handbk.pdf (accessed 2/11/15)

NHS England/P&I/Strategic Systems and Technology (2014) *Open API Architecture Policy.* NHS England, Leeds: https://www.england.nhs.uk/wp-content/uploads/2014/05/open-api-policy.pdf (accessed 22/01/16)

NHS Institute for Innovation and Improvement (2008) *DNAs Reducing Did Not Attends:* http://www.institute.nhs.uk/quality_and_service_improvement_tools/quality_and_service_improvement_tools/dnas_-_reducing_did_not_attends.html (accessed 19/1/16)

National Electrical Manufacturers Association (2015) *DICOM PS3.1 2015c –Introduction and Overview:* http://dicom.nema.org/medical/dicom/current/output/pdf/part01.pdf (accessed 25/12/15)

Nichol PB (2015) *Blockchain Technology: The Solution for Healthcare Interoperability:* https://www.linkedin.com/pulse/blockchain-technology-solution-healthcare-peter-b-nichol (accessed 17/01/16)

Padrez KA, Ungar L, Schwartz HA, *et al.* (2016) Linking social media and medical record data: a study of adults presenting to an academic, urban emergency department. *British Medical Journal Quality and Safety* **25**(6):414–423.

Peel D (2012) *Should Every Patient Have a Unique ID Number for All Medical Records?- No Privacy Would Suffer:* http://www.wsj.com/articles/SB10001424052970204124204577154661814932978 published online 23/12/2012

Ross SE, Todd J, Moore LA, Beaty BL, Wittevrongel L, Lin CT (2005) Expectations of patients and physicians regarding patient-accessible medical records. *Journal of Medical Internet Research* **7**(2):e13.

Royal College of Radiologists (2016) *iRefer:* https://www.rcr.ac.uk/clinical-radiology/being-consultant/rcr-referral-guidelines/about-irefer (accessed 19/1/16)

Suzuki K (2013) Machine Learning in Computer-aided Diagnosis of the Thorax and University Hospital Southampton (2016) *My Health Record*: http://www.uhs.nhs.uk/AboutTheTrust/Myhealthrecord/Myhealthrecord.aspx. (accessed 22/1/2016)

Chapter 7

Al-Hajeri M, Clarke M (2015) Future trends in picture archiving and communication system (PACS). In: *SPIE Medical Imaging*. International Society for Optics and Photonics. pp. 94180K–94180K.

Buabbas AJ, Al-Shamali DA, Sharma P, Haidar S, Al-Shawaf H (2016) Users' perspectives on a picture archiving and communication system (PACS): an in-depth study in a teaching hospital in Kuwait. *JMIR Medical Informatics* **4**(2):e21.

Cooke R (2014) Utilization management and ACR select. *Radiology management* **37**(2):9–12.

Hammana I, Lepanto L, Poder T, Bellemare C, Ly MS (2015) Speech recognition in the radiology department: a systematic review. *Health Information Management Journal* **44**(2):4–10.

Hart JL, Mcbride A, Blunt D, Gishen P, Strickland N (2010) Immediate and sustained benefits of a "total" implementation of speech recognition reporting. *The British Journal of Radiology* **83**(989):424–427.

Jorritsma W, Cnossen F, Dierckx RA, Oudkerk M, Van Ooijen PM (2016) Post-deployment usability evaluation of a radiology workstation. *International Journal of Medical Informatics* **85**(1):28–35.

Joshi V, Narra VR, Joshi K, Lee K, Melson D (2014) PACS administrators' and radiologists' perspective on the importance of features for PACS selection. *Journal of Digital Imaging* **27**(4):486–495.

Keen C (2014) The clinical decision-support mandate: now what? *Radiology Business* July, pp. 1–6.

McGurk S, Brauer K, Macfarlane TV, Duncan KA (2014) The effect of voice recognition software on comparative error rates in radiology reports. *The British Journal of Radiology* **81**(970):767–770.

Mansoori B, Erhard KK, Sunshine JL (2012) Picture archiving and communication system (PACS) implementation, integration & benefits in an integrated health system. *Academic Radiology* **19**(2):229–235.

Nance Jr, JW, Meenan C, Nagy PG (2013) The future of the radiology information system. *American Journal of Roentgenology* **200**(5):1064–1070.

NHS England. *Safer Hospitals Safer Wards – Achieving and Integrated Digital Care Record*: https://www.england.nhs.uk/wp-content/uploads/2013/07/safer-hosp-safer-wards.pdf (accessed 4/10/16)

Pynoo B, Devolder P, Duyck W, van Braak J, Sijnave B, Duyck P (2012) Do hospital physicians' attitudes change during PACS implementation? A cross-sectional acceptance study. *International Journal of Medical Informatics* **81**(2):88–97.

Ringler MD, Goss BC, Bartholmai BJ (2017) Syntactic and semantic errors in radiology reports associated with speech recognition software. *Health Informatics Journal* **23**(1):3–13.

Society and College of Radiographers (2013) *Preliminary Clinical Evaluation and Clinical Reporting by Radiographers: Policy and Practice Guidance.*

Taylor-Phillips S, Grove A, Hoffmeister S, *et al.* (2014) Going 'paperless' in an English National Health Service (NHS) breast cancer screening service: the introduction of fully digital mammography. *Health* **6**(5):468–474.

Chapter 8

ISO 12052:2006 *Health Informatics – Digital Imaging and Communication in Medicine (DICOM) Including Workflow and Data Management.*

National Electrical Manufacturers Association (NEMA). *The DICOM Standard:* http://dicom.nema.org/standard.html

Chapter 9

FHIR – https://www.hl7.org/fhir/

IHE – http://wiki.ihe.net/index.php/Cross-enterprise_Document_Sharing_for_Imaging

Chapter 11

HSCIC (2013). *Clinical Risk Management: its Application in the Deployment and Use of Health IT Systems.* Department of Health.

Chapter 12

Baron RJ, Fabens EL, Schiffman M, Wolf E (2005) Electronic health records: just around the corner? Or over the cliff? *Annals of Internal Medicine* **143**(3):222–226.

Bosanquet D, Cho J, Williams N, Gower D, Thomas KG, Lewis M (2013) Requesting radiological investigations – do junior doctors know their patients? A cross-sectional survey *Journal of the Royal Society of Medicine Short Reports* **4**(1):3.

Franczak MJ, Klein M, Raslau F, Bergholte J, Mark LP, Ulmer JL (2014) In emergency departments, radiologists' access to EHRs may influence interpretations and medical management. *Health Affairs* (Millwood) **33**(5):800–806.

Gates P, Urquhart J (2007) The electronic, 'paperless' medical office; has it arrived? *Internal Medicine Journal* **37**(2):108–11.

Lehnbom EC, Adams K, Day RO, Westbrook JI, Baysari MT (2014) iPad use during ward rounds: an observational study. *Studies in Health Technology and Informatics* **204**:67–73.

Más A, Parra P, Bermejo RM, Hidalgo MD, Calle JE (2016) Improving quality in healthcare: what makes a satisfied patient? *Revista de Calidad Asistencial* **31**(4):196–203.

Rosenfeld KH (2013) Streamlining medical image sharing for continuity of care. *Radiology Management* **35**(6):16–9; quiz 20–1.

Seah MK, Murphy CG, McDonald S, Carrothers A (2016) Incidental findings on whole-body trauma computed tomography: experience at a major trauma centre. *Injury* **47**(3):691–694.

Chapter 13

2015 No. 102 Public Procurement *The Public Contracts Regulations 2015* Directive 2014/24/EU of the European Parliament and of the Council of 26 February 2014 on public procurement and repealing Directive 2004/18/EC.

An Introduction to Public Procurement, Office of Government Commerce Public Contracts Regulations 2015: Requirements on Pre-qualification Questionnaires: https://www.gov.uk/government/publications/public-contracts-regulations-2015-requirements-on-pre-qualification-questionnaires

HM Treasury *The Green Book: Appraisal and Evaluation in Central Government.*

HM Treasury's *Managing Public Money.*

OJEU Directives: http://www.ojeu.eu/directives.aspx

Chapter 14

Access to Health Records Act 1990.

Data Protection Act 1998.

Department of Health (2001) *NHS Confidentiality Code of Practice.*

Department of Health (2013) *The Information Governance Review: To Share or Not to Share.*

Freedom of Information Act 2000.

General Data Protection Regulation (Regulation (EU) 2016/679).

Google Health is Closing (2016) Google Inc: https://googleblog.blogspot.
co.uk/2011/06/update-on-google-health-and-google.html
Information Commissioners Office. *Anonymisation: Managing Data Protection
Risk Code of Practice.*
Ionising Radiation (Medical Exposure) Regulations 2000 (IRMER).
ISB 0129 *Clinical Risk Management: its Application in the Manufacture of
Health IT Systems Version 3* – Specification (2013). NHS Digital.
ISB 0160 *Clinical Risk Management: its Application in the Deployment and Use
of Health IT Systems Version 2* – Specification (2013). NHS Digital.
ISO 22600: 2014 Health informatics: *Privilege Control and Roll Based Access.*
The Caldicott Committee (December 1997). *The Caldicott Report.*
Department of Health.
The Ionising Radiations Regulations 1999.
The National Data Guardian (2016) *Review of Data Security, Consent and
Opt-outs.*

Chapter 15

ISO 31000:2009 *Risk Management – Principles and Guidelines*. International
Organization for Standardization.
Cloud Accountability Project: www.a4Cloud.eu
Cloud Security Alliance: www.CloudSecurityAlliance.org
Failure of core network at Northumbria downs IT systems: https://www.
digitalhealth.net/2017/02/northumbria-network-failure-downs-it-
systems/
Healthcare Information and Management Systems Society: www.himss.org
I.T. Service Management Forum UK: www.itsmf.co.uk
Leeds hospitals surgery postponed after IT problem: http://www.bbc.
co.uk/news/uk-england-leeds-37422613
Managing Successful Projects with PRINCE2® 2009 Edition; (2009). Office
of Government & Commerce (Axelos).
National Institute of Standards and Technology: www.nist.gov

Chapter 16

Bott OJ, Dresing K, Wagner M, Raab BW,Teistler M (2011) Informatics in
radiology: use of a C-Arm fluoroscopy simulator to support training in intraoperative radiography. *Radiographics* **31**(3):E63–75.
Health and Care Professions Council Continuing Professional Development:
http://hpc-uk.org/registrants/cpd/ (accessed 9/6/16)
OsiriX (2014) *About Osirix:* http://www.osirix-viewer.com/AboutOsiriX.
html (accessed 13/6/16)

Oxford University Press (2016) *Learning About Virtual Learning Environments/Course Management System Content:* http://global. oup.com/uk/orc/learnvle/ (accessed 9/6/16)

Royal College of Radiologists (2012) *Picture Archiving and Communication Systems (PACS) and Guidelines on Diagnostic Display Devices.* RCR, London, UK.

Sectra (2015) *Interactive Medical Education:* http://www.sectra.com/medical/sectra_table/ (accessed 10/6/16)

Shaderware (2014) *Radiography Training Using 3D Interactive Simulation:* http://www.shaderware.com/index.html (accessed 10/6/16)

Society of Radiographers (2016) *CPD Now:* https://www.sor.org/learning/cpd/cpd-now (accessed 9/6/16)

University of Bradford (2014) *Bradton:* http://bradton.pbworks.com/w/page/51823092/Home%20Page (accessed 10/6/16)

VERTUAL (2016) *VERT –The Flight Simulator for Linacs:* http://www.vertual.eu/products/vert (accessed 10/6/16)

Chapter 17

NHS Employers (2006) *Pay and Reward: National Profiles for Diagnostic and Therapeutic Radiography.*

NIHR (2013) *National Institute for Health Research Funding Data: Research Project Funding Data.*

Peck A (2013) *Bushcraft: Educating the PACS Team* Proceedings of the UK Radiological Congress, 2013.

Peck A (2013) *CPD for the PACS Team* ePoster UK Radiological Congress.

Peck A, Patel A, Tucker K (in press) *The State of the UK Imaging Informatics Profession.* Society and College of Radiographers.

INDEX

Note: Page numbers in *italic* refer to figures or tables

Index

T - #0125 - 111024 - C248 - 198/129/12 - PB - 9781498763233 - Gloss Lamination